MATHEMATICS IN INDUSTRY   10

Editors
Hans-Georg Bock
Frank de Hoog
Avner Friedman
Arvind Gupta
Helmut Neunzert
William R. Pulleyblank
Torgeir Rusten
Fadil Santosa
Anna-Karin Tornberg

THE EUROPEAN CONSORTIUM
FOR MATHEMATICS IN INDUSTRY

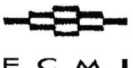

SUBSERIES

Managing Editor
Vincenzo Capasso

Editors
Robert Mattheij
Helmut Neunzert
Otmar Scherzer

Otmar Scherzer

Mathematical Models for Registration and Applications to Medical Imaging

With 54 Figures, 12 in Color, and 12 Tables

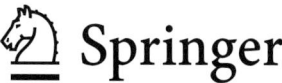

Editor

Otmar Scherzer
Universität Innsbruck
Institut für Informatik, Technikerstr. 21A
A – 6020 Innsbruck, Austria
e-mail: otmar.scherzer@uibk.ac.at

Library of Congress Control Number: 2006926829

Mathematics Subject Classification (2000): 65J15, 65F22, 94a08, 94J40, 94K24

ISBN-10 3-540-25029-8 Springer Berlin Heidelberg New York
ISBN-13 978-3-540-25029-6 Springer Berlin Heidelberg New York

This work is subject to copyright. All rights are reserved, whether the whole or part of the material is concerned, specifically the rights of translation, reprinting, reuse of illustrations, recitation, broadcasting, reproduction on microfilm or in any other way, and storage in data banks. Duplication of this publication or parts thereof is permitted only under the provisions of the German Copyright Law of September 9, 1965, in its current version, and permission for use must always be obtained from Springer. Violations are liable for prosecution under the German Copyright Law.

Springer is a part of Springer Science+Business Media

springer.com

© Springer-Verlag Berlin Heidelberg 2006
Printed in Germany

The use of general descriptive names, registered names, trademarks, etc. in this publication does not imply, even in the absence of a specific statement, that such names are exempt from the relevant protective laws and regulations and therefore free for general use.

Typeset by the editors & SPI Publisher Services
Production: LE-TEX Jelonek, Schmidt & Vöckler GbR, Leipzig
Cover design: *design & production* GmbH, Heidelberg
Printed on acid-free paper   SPIN: 11397403   46/3100/SPI - 5 4 3 2 1 0

Preface

Image registration is an emerging topic in image processing with many applications in medical imaging, picture and movie processing. The classical problem of image registration is concerned with finding an appropriate transformation between two data sets. This fuzzy definition of registration requires a mathematical modeling and in particular a mathematical specification of the terms *appropriate* transformations and *correlation* between data sets. Depending on the type of application, typically Euler, rigid, plastic, elastic deformations are considered. The variety of similarity measures ranges from a simple L^p distance between the pixel values of the data to mutual information or entropy distances.

This goal of this book is to highlight by some experts in industry and medicine relevant and emerging image registration applications and to show new emerging mathematical technologies in these areas.

Currently, many registration application are solved based on variational principle requiring sophisticated analysis, such as calculus of variations and the theory of partial differential equations, to name but a few. Due to the numerical complexity of registration problems efficient numerical realization are required. Concepts like multi-level solver for partial differential equations, non-convex optimization, and so on play an important role. Mathematical and numerical issues in the area of registration are discussed by some of the experts in this volume.

Moreover, the importance of registration for industry and medical imaging is discussed from a medical doctor and from a manufacturer point of view.

We would like to thank Stephanie Schimkowitsch for a marvelous job in typesetting this manuscript. Moreover, we would like to thank Prof. Vincenzo Capasso for the continuous encouragement and support of this book and I would like to express my thanks to Ute McCrory (Springer) for her patience during the preparation of the manuscript.

The work of myself is supported by the FWF, Austria Science Foundation, Projects Y-123INF, FSP 9203-N12 and FSP 9207-N12. Without the support of the FWF for my research this volume would not be possible.

June, 2005 *Otmar Scherzer (Innsbruck)*

Table of Contents

Part I Numerical Methods

A Generalized Image Registration Framework using Incomplete Image Information – with Applications to Lesion Mapping
Stefan Henn, Lars Hömke, Kristian Witsch 3

Medical Image Registration and Interpolation by Optical Flow with Maximal Rigidity
Stephen L. Keeling 27

Registration of Histological Serial Sectionings
Jan Modersitzki, Oliver Schmitt, and Stefan Wirtz 63

Computational Methods for Nonlinear Image Registration
Ulrich Clarenz, Marc Droske, Stefan Henn, Martin Rumpf, Kristian Witsch ... 81

A Survey on Variational Optic Flow Methods for Small Displacements
Joachim Weickert, Andrés Bruhn, Thomas Brox, and Nils Papenberg 103

Part II Applications

Fast Image Matching for Generation of Panorama Ultrasound
Armin Schoisswohl 139

Inpainting of Movies Using Optical Flow
Harald Grossauer 151

Part III Medical Applications

Multimodality Registration in Daily Clinical Practice
Reto Bale 165

Colour Images
Clarenz et al., Henn et al., Weickert et al., Bale 185

List of Contributors

Otmar Scherzer
University of Innsbruck
Institute of Computer Science
Technikerstraße 21a
6020 Innsbruck, Austria
otmar.scherzer@uibk.ac.at

Armin Schoisswohl
GE Medical Systems
Kretz Ultrasound
Tiefenbach 15
4871 Zipf, Austria
armin.schoisswohl@med.ge.com

Reto Bale
Universitätsklinik für Radiodiagnostik
SIP-Labor
Anichstraße 35
6020 Innsbruck, Austria
reto.bale@uibk.ac.at

Harald Grossauer
University of Innsbruck
Institute of Computer Science
Technikerstraße 21a
6020 Innsbruck, Austria
harald.grossauer@uibk.ac.at

Stefan Henn
Heinrich-Heine University of Düsseldorf
Lehrstuhl für Mathematische Optimierung
Mathematisches Institut
Universitätsstraße 1
40225 Düsseldorf, Germany
henn@am.uni-duesseldorf.de

Lars Hömke
Forschungszentrum Jülich GmbH
Institut für Medizin
Street No.
52425 Jülich, Germany
hoemke@am.uni-duesseldorf.de

Kristian Witsch
Heinrich-Heine University of Düsseldorf
Lehrstuhl für Angewandte Mathematik
Mathematisches Institut
Universitätsstraße 1
40225 Düsseldorf, Germany
witsch@am.uni-duesseldorf.de

Stephen L. Keeling
Karl-Franzens University of Graz
Institute of Mathematics
Heinrichstraße 36
8010 Graz, Austria
stephen.keeling@uni-graz.ac.at

Jan Modersitzki
University of Lübeck
Institute of Mathematics
Wallstraße 40
D-23560 Lübeck
modersitzki@math.uni-luebeck.de

Oliver Schmitt
University of Rostock

Institute of Anatomy
Gertrudenstraße 9
D-18055 Rostock, Germany
schmitt@med.uni-rostock.de

Stefan Wirtz
University of Lübeck
Institute of Mathematics
Wallstraße 40
D-23560 Lübeck
wirtz@math.uni-luebeck.de

Ulrich Clarenz
Gerhard-Mercator University of Duisburg
Institute of Mathematics
Lotharstraße 63/65,
47048 Duisburg, Germany
clarenz@math.uni-duisburg.de

Marc Droske
University of California
Math Sciences Department
520 Portola Plaza,
Los Angeles, CA, 90055, USA
droske@math.ucla.edu

Stefan Henn
Heinrich-Heine University of Düsseldorf
Lehrstuhl für Mathematische Optimierung
Universitätsstraße 1
40225 Düsseldorf, Germany
henn@am.uni-duesseldorf.de

Martin Rumpf
Rheinische Friedrich-Wilhelms-Universität Bonn
Institut für Numerische Simulation
Nussallee 15,
53115 Bonn, Germany
martin.rumpf@ins.uni-bonn.de

Kristian Witsch
Heinrich-Heine University of Düsseldorf
Lehrstuhl für Angewandte Mathematik
Universitätsstraße 1
40225 Düsseldorf, Germany
witsch@math.uni-duisburg.de

Joachim Weickert
Mathematical Image Analysis Group,
Faculty of Mathematics and Computer Science,
Saarland University, Building 27,
66041 Saarbrücken, Germany.
weickert@mia.uni-saarland.de.

Andrés Bruhn
Mathematical Image Analysis Group,
Faculty of Mathematics and Computer Science,
Saarland University, Building 27,
66041 Saarbrücken, Germany.
bruhn@mia.uni-saarland.de.

Nils Papenberg
Mathematical Image Analysis Group,
Faculty of Mathematics and Computer Science,
Saarland University, Building 27,
66041 Saarbrücken, Germany.
papenberg@mia.uni-saarland.de.

Thomas Brox
Mathematical Image Analysis Group,
Faculty of Mathematics and Computer Science,
Saarland University, Building 27,
66041 Saarbrücken, Germany.
brox@mia.uni-saarland.de.

Part I

Numerical Methods

A Generalized Image Registration Framework using Incomplete Image Information – with Applications to Lesion Mapping

Stefan Henn[1], Lars Hömke[2], and Kristian Witsch[3]

[1] Lehrstuhl für Mathematische Optimierung, Mathematisches Institut, Heinrich-Heine Universität Düsseldorf, Universitätsstraße 1, D-40225 Düsseldorf, Germany.
henn@am.uni-duesseldorf.de
[2] Institut für Medizin, Forschungszentrum Jülich GmbH,
D-52425 Jülich, Germany. hoemke@am.uni-duesseldorf.de
[3] Lehrstuhl für Angewandte Mathematik, Mathematisches Institut, Heinrich-Heine Universität Düsseldorf, Universitätsstraße 1, D-40225 Düsseldorf, Germany.
witsch@am.uni-duesseldorf.de

Abstract This paper presents a novel variational approach to obtain a d-dimensional displacement field $u = (u_1, \cdots, u_d)^t$, which matches two images with incomplete information. A suitable energy, which effectively measures the similarity between the images is proposed. An algorithm, which efficiently finds the displacement field by minimizing the associated energy is presented. In order to compensate the absence of image information, the approach is based on an energy minimizing interpolation of the displacement field into the holes of missing image data. This interpolation is computed via a gradient descent flow with respect to an auxiliary energy norm. This incorporates smoothness constraints into the displacement field. Applications of the presented technique include the registration of damaged histological sections and registration of brain lesions to a reference atlas. We conclude the paper by a number of examples of these applications.

Keywords image registration, inpainting, functional minimization, finite difference discretization, regularization, multi-scale

1 Introduction.

Deformable image registration of brain images has been an active topic of research in recent years. Driven by ever more powerful computers, image registration algorithms have become important tools, e.g. in

– guidance of surgery,
– diagnostics,
– quantitative analysis of brain structures (interhemispheric, interareal and interindividual),
– ontogenetic differences between cortical areas,
– interindividual brain studies.

The need for registration in interindividual brain studies arises from the fact that the human brain exhibits a high interindividual variability. While the topology is stable on the level of primary structures, not only the general shape, but also the spatial localization of brain structures varies considerably across brains. That renders a direct comparison impossible. Hence, brains have to be registered to a common "reference space", i.e. they are registered to a reference brain. Often there are also, so-called maps, that reside in the same reference space. In so called brain atlases there are additional maps that contain different kinds of information about the reference brain, such as labeled cortical regions. Once an individual brain has been registered to the reference brain the maps can be transferred to the registered brain. It is not only that obtaining the information from the individual brain itself is often more intricate than registering it to a reference, in some cases it is also impossible. For instance, the microstructure of the brain cannot be analyzed in vivo, since the resolution of in vivo imaging methods, such as MRI and PET, is too low. Registration can also be a means of creating such maps, by transferring information from different brains into a reference space.

In the last decade computational algorithms have been developed in order to map two images, i.e. to determine a "best fit" between them. Although these techniques have been applied very successfully for both the uni- and the multi-modal case (e.g. see [1, 2, 7, 8, 10, 11, 13, 19, 21, 22, 25]) these techniques may be less appropriate for studies using brain-damaged subjects, since there is no compensation for the structural distortion introduced by a lesion (e.g. a tumor, ventricular enlargement, large regions of atypical pixel intensity values, etc.).

Generally the computed solution cannot be trusted in the area of a lesion. The magnitude of the effect on the solution depends on the character of the registration scheme employed. It is not only that these effects are undesirable, but also that in some cases one is especially interested in where the lesion would be in the other image. If, for instance, we want to know which function is usually performed by the damaged area, we could register the lesioned brain to an atlas and map the lesion to functional data within the reference space.

In more general terms the problem can be phrased as follows. Given are two images and a domain G including a segmentation of the lesions. The aim of the proposed image registration algorithm is to find a "smooth" displacement field, which

– minimizes a given similarity functional and
– conserve the lesion in the transformed template image.

There have been approaches to register lesions manually[12]. In this paper we present a novel automatically image registration approach for human brain volumes with structural distortions (e.g a lesion). The main idea is to define a suitable matching energy, which effectively measures the similarity between the images. Since the minimization solely the matching energy is an ill-posed problem we minimize the energy by a gradient descent flow with respect to a regularity energy borrowed from linear elasticity theory. The regularization energy incorporates smoothness constraints into the displacement field during the iteration.

The presented approach can be seen as the well known "image inpainting approach" (e.g. see [3, 5, 6]) for the unknown displacement field u. In inpainting missing or damaged parts of an image are restored using information from the surrounding area. Applications include the restoration of damaged photographs and movies or the removal of selected objects.

The analogy to image inpainting is given as follows: both approaches

1. consider a data model restricted on a domain $\Omega \setminus G$, where data is missing on G,
2. use a regularity energy defined on Ω,
3. determine a solution defined on Ω.

	Inpainting	proposed appr.
Input:	$I\|_{\Omega \setminus G}$	$T\|_{\Omega \setminus G_1}, R\|_{\Omega \setminus G_2}$
Data model:	restricted $\Omega \setminus G$	restricted $\Omega \setminus (G_1 \cup G_2)$
Regularity energy:	defined on Ω	defined on Ω
Output:	entire image $I\|_\Omega$	entire displacement field $u\|_\Omega$

The paper is organized as follows. In section 2 we describe an abstract mathematical framework to handle a variety of distance measures so-called matching energies. In the next section we present a novel variational approach, which matches two images with absent information on a part of the image-domain. The aim of the approach is to obtain a d-dimensional displacement field defined on Ω which preserves the lesion in the transformed images.

For this reason a suitable matching energy, which effectively measures the similarity between the images is proposed. Even when the images contain complete information, the sole minimization of the matching energy is an ill-posed problem. Thus, we add an auxiliary Lagrange term, given by an energy norm, which incorporates smoothness constraints into the displacement field.

In order to present a general description of the approach we use a general framework up to this point. In section 4 we present the numerical description, with a particular choice of the matching energy as well as for the energy norm for the displacement field. We discuss the discretization of the problem and the underlying numerical scheme to solve the resulting subproblems. In section 5 we present two- and three-dimensional results, where brain data is used. For the two-dimensional example we use a digitized histological section. In the three-dimensional case the approach is applied to lesioned MR volume data that is registered to a reference brain.

2 Abstract Framework.

Given are two images, a reference R and a template T using the same or different imaging modalities. We assume that in continuous variables the images can be represented by compactly supported functions

$$T, R : \Omega \subset \mathbb{R}^d \to \mathbb{R}.$$

Usually, these images are two- or three-dimensional. This means, the map associates with each pixel (picture element)

$$x = (x_1, \cdots, x_d)^t$$

on the image domain Ω its intensities $T(x)$ and $R(x)$. For the purpose of numerical computation Ω will simply be the d-dimensional unit square $[0,1]^d$. We assume that T is distorted by an invertible deformation ϕ^{-1}. We search for a transformation

$$\phi(u)(\cdot) : \mathbb{R}^d \to \mathbb{R}^d, \quad \phi(u)(x) : x \mapsto (x_1 - u_1(x), \cdots, x_d - u_d(x))^t$$

that depends on the unknown displacements

$$u : \mathbb{R}^d \to \mathbb{R}^d, \quad u : x \mapsto u(x) := (u_1(x), \cdots, u_d(x))^t.$$

The goal of image registration is to determine $u(x)$ in such a way that the transformed template $T \circ \phi(u(x))$ matches the reference R. The image registration problem can be identified with a minimization problem in the following manner:

Problem 1. IMAGE REGISTRATION PROBLEM
For an energy functional

$$D[R, T, \Omega; u(x)] := \int_\Omega \Phi(R, T, u) \, dx \; : \; \mathbb{R}^d \to \mathbb{R},$$

which measures the disparity between $T \circ \phi(u(x))$ and $R(x)$ on the image domain Ω, the image registration problem is given by the following minimization problem:

$$\text{Find } u(x), \text{ such that } D[R, T, \Omega; u(x)] \text{ is minimal.} \tag{1}$$

Thus we ask for solutions of the problem to minimize $D[R, T, \Omega; u(x)]$ over

$$L_2^d(\Omega) := \underbrace{L_2(\Omega) \times \cdots \times L_2(\Omega)}_{d-times}.$$

A minimizer $u(x)$ of (1) is characterized by the necessary condition

$$grad\big(D[R, T, u(x)]\big) = 0,$$

where $grad\big(D[R, T, u(x)]\big) \in L_2^d(\Omega)$. Indeed, we require

$$\langle grad(D[R, T, u(x)]), \varphi \rangle = 0 \quad \forall \varphi \in L_2^d(\Omega).$$

In the following we denote the so-called external forces $grad\big(D[R, T, u(x)]\big)$ just by $f(u(x))$. In the image registration process the task of the external forces is to bring similar regions of the images into correspondence. For instance, in the situation that the intensities of the given images are comparable, a common approach is to minimize their squared difference (see, e.g. [1, 2, 7, 13, 21]) for all $x \in \Omega$, i.e. to minimize

$$D_{SD}[R,T;\ u(x)] = \int_{\Omega} \Big(T(x_1 - u_1(x), \cdots, x_d - u_d(x)) - R(x_1, \cdots, x_d)\Big)^2 d\Omega. \tag{2}$$

It is used, for example, in the case that the images are recorded with the same imaging machinery, the so-called mono-modal image registration. The necessary condition for a minimizer $u^*(x)$ of (2) is given by:

$$f_{SD}(u(x)) = -grad\big(T(x_1 - u_1(x), \cdots, x_d - u_d(x))\big) \cdot \\ \big(T(x_1 - u_1(x), \cdots, x_d - u_d(x)) - R(x_1, \cdots, x_d)\big)$$

see, e.g. [20].

Another kind of problem is the so-called multimodality image matching (see, e.g. [9, 22, 23, 26, 29]). Here, the distance between the images is measured by mutual information or entropy based functionals.

Recently, an approach based on the definition of a matching energy, which measures the local morphological "defect" between the images, has been presented [11].

Unfortunately, the image registration problem (1) is not well posed: Solutions, if they exist, are in general neither unique nor stable. Different solutions can give very similar outputs, and small data errors can yield very different solutions. Therefore, the approximations u of (1) may be useless. One has to define better approximate solutions. Since the problem is ill-posed, we have to apply a regularizing technique to solve the problem in a stable way. Many regularization methods are discussed in the literature and the choice of the regularization term depends crucially on the underlying application.

3 Gradient Descent Flow Using Incomplete Image Information.

The aim of this section is to determine a displacement field u on domains where the image information is unavailable.

3.1 Extension of the Similarity Functional

Let Ω denote the complete image domain for the image registration problem presented in the previous section. We assume that there are domains $U_i \subset \Omega$, $1 \leq i \leq s$, where image data in the template image T is missing respectively domains $V_j \subset \Omega$, $1 \leq j \leq t$, where image data in the reference image R is missing.

Then the image registration problem is given by:

> **Problem 2.** IMAGE REGISTRATION WITH INCOMPLETE INFORMATION
> Let $G := G_U \cup G_V$ and $\Omega' = \Omega \setminus G$ an open domain, with
> $$G_U = \left\{ x \in \mathbb{R}^d \mid x \in \Omega \cap (U_1 \cup \cdots \cup U_s) \right\}$$
> and
> $$G_V = \left\{ x \in \mathbb{R}^d \mid x \in \Omega \cap (V_1 \cup \cdots \cup V_t) \right\}.$$
> Then the complete image registration problem for images with incomplete information is given by the following minimization problem:
> $$\text{Find } u(x), \text{ such that } D[R, T, \Omega'; u] \text{ is minimal.} \qquad (3)$$

In order to solve the problem we define an extension of the functional D as follows.

Definition 1. *The* **zero extension** $D_\epsilon[R, T, \Omega'; u]$ *of the similarity function is defined by*
$$D_\epsilon[R, T, \Omega'; u] := \int_{\Omega'} \Phi_\epsilon(R, T, u) \, dx,$$
with
$$\Phi_\epsilon(R, T, u) := \begin{cases} \Phi_\epsilon(R, T, u) & \text{if } x \in \Omega', \\ 0 & \text{if } x \in G. \end{cases}$$

With this definition we can restate problem 2.

> **Problem 3.** MODIFIED IMAGE REGISTRATION PROBLEM
> By using the zero extension of the similarity function $D_\epsilon[R, T, \Omega; u]$ the complete image registration problem for images with incomplete information is given by the following minimization problem:
> $$\text{Find } u(x), \text{ such that } D_\epsilon[R, T, \Omega; u] \text{ is minimal.} \qquad (4)$$

We now describe an approach to solve the minimization problem. Because the problem is nonlinear, we have to use an iterative method. Assume that after k iterations a current deformation $\phi_k = x - u^{(k)}(x)$ is given, then the domains G and Ω'_k are changed in the following way

$$G_k = \phi_k(G_U) \cup G_V, \quad \Omega'_k = \Omega \setminus G_k,$$

since the displacements only acts on the template image.

3.2 Extended Iterative Minimization Method

To minimize $D_\epsilon[R, T, \Omega; u]$ for a given current approximation $u^{(k)}$, we search for an approximation $u^{(k+1)}$ so that

$$D_\epsilon[R, T, \Omega; u^{(k+1)}] < D_\epsilon[R, T, \Omega; u^{(k)}].$$

The reduction for the next iterate $u^{(k+1)}$ is given approximately by

$$D_\epsilon[R, T, \Omega; u^{(k+1)}] - D_\epsilon[R, T, \Omega; u^{(k)}] \approx \frac{\partial}{\partial d^{(k)}} D_\epsilon[R, T, \Omega; u^{(k)}], \quad (5)$$

where the Gâtaux-derivative at $u^{(k)}$ in the descend direction

$$d^{(k)} = u^{(k+1)} - u^{(k)}$$

is given by

$$\frac{\partial}{\partial d^{(k)}} D_\epsilon[R, T, \Omega; u^{(k)}] = \left\langle f_k, d^{(k)} \right\rangle_{L_2(\Omega)}$$

with

$$f_k := f(u^{(k)}) = \begin{cases} grad(D_\epsilon[R, T, \Omega; u^{(k)}]) & \text{if } x \in \Omega'_k, \\ 0 & \text{if } x \in G_k. \end{cases}$$

By using the negative gradient the nonlinear steepest descent iteration for problem 3 is given by

$$u^{(k+1)} = u^{(k)} - \tau_k f_k, \quad (6)$$

with

$$\tau_k = \arg\min_{\tau \in \mathbb{R}} D_\epsilon[R, T, \Omega; u^{(k)} - \tau f_k].$$

Unfortunately, for most real applications the steepest descent iteration (6) is not suitable to solve the image registration problem. This is at least due to two factors. First, because of the ill-posedness, this method does not have global convergence properties. Second, due to noise sensitivity of the ill-posed registration problem, regularization techniques have to be applied in order to compute meaningful solutions. Hence, to ensure robustness and fast local convergence it is necessary to incorporate additional information.

3.3 Filling-in by an Unified Regularization Approach

A natural way to alleviate this effects is to find a descend direction subject to an energy constraint $|| \cdot ||_E$ smaller than some particular value η, i.e.

$$\arg\min \left\langle f_k, d^{(k)} \right\rangle_{L_2(\Omega)}, \quad \text{s.t.} \quad ||d^{(k)}||_E^2 \leq \eta,$$

where the energy norm $|| \cdot ||_E$ is defined by

$$||v||_E = \sqrt{\langle v, v \rangle_E}$$

with inner product

$$\langle v, w \rangle_E = \langle Lv, w \rangle_{L_2^d(\Omega)}$$

and a symmetric positive definite operator L.

Remark 1. In order to guarantee positive definiteness of the operator L in the following, we assume Dirichlet boundary conditions, i.e.

$$d^{(k)}(x) = 0 \quad \text{for} \quad x \in \partial\Omega \quad \text{and} \quad k = 0, 1, 2, \cdots.$$

Other possibilities to guarantee positive definiteness are described in cf. [17].

The method of Lagrange multipliers gives the functional

$$\arg\min_{d^{(k)}} \left\{ \langle f_k, d^{(k)} \rangle_{L_2(\Omega)} + \alpha \langle Ld^{(k)}, d^{(k)} \rangle_{L_2(\Omega)} \right\}, \tag{7}$$

with some parameter $\alpha(\eta) = \alpha > 0$. We have the following result:

Theorem 1. *The unique minimizer of (7) is characterized by the following boundary value problem*

$$\left. \begin{array}{ll} \alpha L\, d^{(k)}(x) = -grad(D_\epsilon[R,T,\Omega;\, u^{(k)}]) & \text{for } x \in \Omega'_k, \\ \alpha L\, d^{(k)}(x) = 0 & \text{for } x \in G_k, \\ d^{(k)}(x) = 0 & \text{for } x \in \partial\Omega. \end{array} \right\} \tag{8}$$

Proof. Since L is a symmetric positive definite operator, a weak solution of (7) is given by the variational equation

$$\langle \alpha Ld^{(k)}, \varphi \rangle_{L_2(\Omega)} = \langle -f_k, \varphi \rangle_{L_2(\Omega)} \tag{9}$$

for every φ with $\varphi = 0$ on $\partial\Omega$. Classical solutions fulfill

$$\alpha L\, d^{(k)}(x) = -f_k \quad \text{for } x \in \Omega,$$
$$d^{(k)}(x) = 0 \quad \text{for } x \in \partial\Omega$$

or equivalent

$$\alpha L\, d^{(k)}(x) = -grad(D_\epsilon[R,T,\Omega;\, u^{(k)}]) \quad \text{for } x \in \Omega'_k,$$
$$\alpha L\, d^{(k)}(x) = 0 \quad \text{for } x \in G_k,$$
$$d^{(k)}(x) = 0 \quad \text{for } x \in \partial\Omega.$$

□

We minimize $D_\epsilon[R,T,\Omega;\, u]$ by successively determining $d^{(k)} = -\alpha^{-1}L^{-1}f_k$ as solution of (8) and perform the following iteration

$$u^{(k+1)} = u^{(k)} + d^{(k)} = u^{(k)} - \alpha^{-1}L^{-1}f_k \quad \text{for } k = 0, 1, \ldots$$

with an initial guess $u^{(0)}(x) = u^*(x)$ and $u^{(k+1)}(x) = 0$ for $x \in \partial\Omega$. If in each iteration step the scalar α^{-1} is chosen to minimize

$$\tau_k = \arg\min_{\alpha^{-1}\in\mathbb{R}} D_\epsilon[R, T, \Omega;\ u^{(k)} - \alpha^{-1}L^{-1}f_k],$$

then one obtains the steepest descent method with respect to the energy $||\cdot||_E^2$. If one restricts the parameter $\alpha^{-1} \in [0, 2||d^{(k)}||_\infty^{-1}]$, i.e.

$$\tau_k = \arg\min_{\alpha^{-1}\in[0,2||d^{(k)}||_\infty^{-1}]} D_\epsilon[R, T, \Omega;\ u^{(k)} - \alpha^{-1}L^{-1}f_k]$$

$$= \arg\min_{\alpha^{-1}\in[0,2]} D_\epsilon[R, T, \Omega;\ u^{(k)} - \alpha^{-1}L^{-1}f_k||d^{(k)}||_\infty^{-1}] \quad (10)$$

one obtains a method known as Landweber iteration with trust-region restriction. This means that the template image is moved in one iteration step by at most two pixels. In practice, this seems to be a reasonable compromise between convergence speed and robustness. We stop the iteration when $grad(D_\epsilon[R, T, \Omega;\ u^{(k)}]) \approx 0$ and get algorithm 1.

Algorithm 1 Iterative minimization of $D_\epsilon[R, T, \Omega;\ u]$

$k = 0;\ u^{(0)} = 0;$
repeat
    calculate $f(u^{(k)}(x))$ on $\Omega'_k = \Omega \setminus G_k$
    compute $d^{(k)}$ from *(8)*
    set $s^{(k)} = d^{(k)}/||d^{(k)}||_\infty$
    compute τ_k by solving problem *(10)*
    set $u^{(k+1)} = u^{(k)} + \tau_k \cdot s^{(k)}$
    set $k = k + 1$
    compute $G_k = \phi_k(G_U) \cup G_V$
until $||f(u^{(k)}(x))||^2 \leq eps$

Remark 2. In some applications it is useful to determine a descent direction subject to a semi-norm. Then the operator L is only positive semi-definite and consequently the operator contains a non-trivial kernel. In this situation one has to consider the following situations:

1. If $f_k \notin (L)$ then
$$\tilde{d}^{(k)} = L^+ f_k$$
is the least squares solution of (8).
2. If $f_k \in (L)$ then all solutions of (8) are given by $d^{(k)} = \tilde{d}^{(k)} + v\lambda$, where $\lambda \in \mathbb{R}^d$ and v is an arbitrary basis for $ker(L)$.

In the second case the parameter λ is chosen to minimize

$$D_\epsilon[R, T, \Omega;\ u^{(k+1)} - \lambda v]$$

in each iteration.

4 Algorithmic Aspects

In this section we will turn to the numerical aspects of the proposed approach. We present an algorithm for the efficient and robust computation of solutions $d^{(k)}$ of (8).

4.1 Model

For our specific application we choose

$$D_\epsilon[T, R, \Omega; u] := \frac{1}{2} \int_{\Omega'} (T(x - u(x)) - R(x))^2 dx \tag{11}$$

as the energy functional, i.e. the least squared difference. For the regularization term $\langle Lu, u \rangle$ we chose the elliptic differential Navier-Lamé operator

$$Lu := -\mu \Delta u - (\mu + \lambda)\nabla(\nabla u), \tag{12}$$

with Dirichlet boundary conditions, i.e. $u = 0$ for $x \in \Gamma$. The "external force" is then given by

$$f(u(x)) = \begin{cases} -\nabla T(x - u(x))\, (T(x - u(x)) - R(x)) \,, x \in \Omega' \\ 0 \hspace{5cm}, \text{otherwise} \end{cases}. \tag{13}$$

4.2 Discretization

For the discretization of the domain $\Omega = [0,1]^d \in \mathbb{R}^d$ we define a grid

$$\mathcal{G}_h^d := \{(x_{1,i_1}, x_{2,i_2}, \ldots, x_{d,i_d}) |\ x_{l,i_j} = i_j \cdot h_l,\ i_j = 0, \ldots, n_l - 1\ j, l = 1, \ldots, d\},$$

with $h_l = 1/(n_l - 1)$. Then the inner points of the discrete domain are

$$\Omega_h^d = \{(x_{1,i_1}, x_{2,i_2}, \ldots, x_{d,i_d}) |\ 1 \leq i_j \leq n_j - 2,\ j = 1, \ldots, d\},$$

and the set of discrete boundary points is defined by

$$\partial \Omega_h^d := \Gamma_h^d = \{(x_{1,i_1}, x_{2,i_2}, \ldots, x_{d,i_d}) |\ \exists j : i_j \in \{0, n_j - 1\}\}.$$

We can also write

$$\Omega_h^d = \mathcal{G}_h^d \cap \Omega^d,$$
$$\partial \Omega_h^d = \Gamma_h^d = \mathcal{G}_h^d \cap \Gamma^d.$$

For G_k we have

$$G_{h,k}^d := \Omega_h^d \cap (G_k \cup \mathcal{U}(G_k)),$$
$$\Omega_h^{'d} := \Omega_h^d \setminus G_{h,k}^d,$$

where $\mathcal{U}$ is a set of points in the neighborhood of G_k which depends on the discrete approximation of external force $f(u(x))$. Specifically $\mathcal{U}(G_k)$ has to be chosen such that there exists no $x = (x_{1,i_1}, \ldots, x_{d,i_d})$ used in the discrete approximation of $f(u(x))$ that is in $\Omega_h^d \cap G_k$.

A Mathematical Image Registration Model with Incomplete Image Information

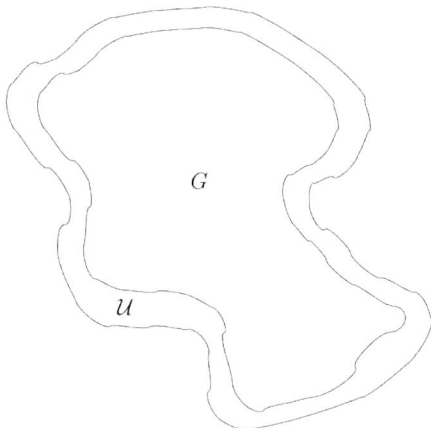

Fig. 1. Depending on the approximation G_k has to be enlarged by $\mathcal{U}$ to avoid that points in G_k are used in the approximation of f.

Example 1. When only the direct neighbors are involved in the discrete approximation of $f(u(x))$, then we have

$$\mathcal{U} := \{x|\ x \pm e_j \cdot h \in G,\ x \in \Omega',\ 1 \leq j \leq d\}.$$

We shall see that this is exactly the case for the approximation that is introduced in the following sections.

For $x \in \bar{\Omega}_h^d$ and $u(x)$ we define the following alternative notation:

$$(x_{1,i_1}, x_{2,i_2}, \ldots, x_{d,i_d})^t \stackrel{\wedge}{=} x_{i_1 i_2 \ldots i_d},$$
$$u(x_{i_1 i_2 \ldots i_d}) \stackrel{\wedge}{=} u_{i_1 i_2 \ldots i_d}.$$

4.3 Approximation

From (12) and (13) we obtain the system of partial differential equations

$$-\mu \left(\sum_{j=1}^{d} \frac{\partial^2 u_i}{\partial x_j^2} \right) - (\lambda + \mu) \frac{\partial}{\partial x_i} \left(\sum_{j=1}^{d} \frac{\partial u_j}{\partial x_j} \right) = f_i(u), \quad i = 1, \ldots, d, \quad (14)$$

where

$$f_i(u) = \begin{cases} (T(x - u(x)) - R(x)) \frac{\partial}{\partial x_i} T(x - u(x)) \text{, for } x \in \Omega_h'^d \\ 0 \qquad\qquad\qquad\qquad\qquad\qquad\qquad\quad \text{, otherwise} \end{cases}. \quad (15)$$

Higher order terms of the Jacobian $J(x - u(x))$ have been omitted, i.e. $J(x - u(x))$ has been replaced by the identity. The partial derivatives are approximated using the finite differences approximations

$$\frac{\partial u_j(x)}{\partial x_l} = \frac{u_j(x+e_l h_l) - u_j(x-e_l h_l)}{2h_l} + \mathcal{O}(h_l^2),$$

$$\frac{\partial^2 u_j(x)}{\partial x_l^2} = \frac{u_j(x+e_l h_l) - 2u_j(x) + u_j(x-e_l h_l)}{h_l^2} + \mathcal{O}(h_l^2),$$

$$\frac{\partial^2 u_j(x)}{\partial x_l \partial x_m} = \frac{1}{4h_l h_m}\Big[u_j(x-e_l h_l - e_m h_m) - u_j(x+e_l h_l - e_m h_m)$$

$$-u_j(x-e_l h_l + e_m h_m) + u_j(x+e_l h_l + e_m h_m)\Big] + \mathcal{O}(\max(h_l, h_m)^2).$$

In the following we give the explicit discretization of the three dimensional case ($d = 3$). Furthermore we will assume $n_l = n$, $l = 1, \ldots, d$. With the short notation defined in section 4.2 we have

$$\frac{\partial u_j}{\partial x_1} \approx \frac{u_{j_{i_1+1,i_2,i_3}} - u_{j_{i_1-1,i_2,i_3}}}{2h},$$

$$\frac{\partial^2 u_j}{\partial x_1^2} \approx \frac{u_{j_{i_1+1,i_2,i_3}} - 2u_{j_{i_1,i_2,i_3}} + u_{j_{i_1-1,i_2,i_3}}}{h^2},$$

$$\frac{\partial^2 u_j}{\partial x_1 \partial x_2} \approx \frac{u_{j_{i_1-1,i_2-1,i_3}} - u_{j_{i_1+1,i_2-1,i_3}} - u_{j_{i_1-1,i_2+1,i_3}} + u_{j_{i_1+1,i_2+1,i_3}}}{4h^2}.$$

These equation can be rewritten in operator form as

$$\frac{\partial u_i}{\partial x_1} \approx \frac{1}{2h}\left[[0]\begin{bmatrix}-1 & 0 & 1\end{bmatrix}[0]\right] u_i,$$

$$\frac{\partial^2 u_i}{\partial x_1^2} \approx \frac{1}{h^2}\left[[0]\begin{bmatrix}1 & -2 & 1\end{bmatrix}[0]\right] u_i,$$

$$\frac{\partial^2 u_i}{\partial x_1 \partial x_2} \approx \frac{1}{4h^2}\left[[0]\begin{bmatrix}1 & 0 & -1\\ 0 & 0 & 0\\ -1 & 0 & 1\end{bmatrix}[0]\right] u_i,$$

$$\Delta_h u_i \approx \sum_{l=1}^{3} \frac{\partial^2 u_i}{\partial x_l^2} = \frac{1}{h^2}\left[[1]\begin{bmatrix}0 & 1 & 0\\ 1 & -6 & 1\\ 0 & 1 & 0\end{bmatrix}[1]\right] u_i$$

where the left and right inner brackets account for the third dimension. For the system of partial differential equation we get

A Mathematical Image Registration Model with Incomplete Image Information

$$f(u) = \begin{cases} -\left(\mu\Delta_h + \frac{\mu+\lambda}{h^2}\left[[0]\begin{bmatrix}1 & -2 & 1\end{bmatrix}[0]\right]\right)u_1 \\ \quad -\frac{(\mu+\lambda)}{4h^2}\left(\left[[0]\begin{bmatrix}1 & 0 & -1\\0 & 0 & 0\\-1 & 0 & 1\end{bmatrix}[0]\right]u_2 + \left[\begin{bmatrix}1 & 0 & -1\end{bmatrix}[0]\begin{bmatrix}-1 & 0 & 1\end{bmatrix}\right]u_3\right) \\[1em] \hline \\ -\frac{(\mu+\lambda)}{4h^2}\left[[0]\begin{bmatrix}1 & 0 & -1\\0 & 0 & 0\\1 & 0 & -1\end{bmatrix}[0]\right]u_1 - \left(\mu\Delta_h + \frac{\mu+\lambda}{h^2}\left[[0]\begin{bmatrix}1\\-2\\1\end{bmatrix}[0]\right]\right)u_2 \\ \quad -\frac{(\mu+\lambda)}{4h^2}\left[[0]\begin{bmatrix}1 & 0 & -1\\0 & 0 & 0\\-1 & 0 & 1\end{bmatrix}[0]\right]u_3 \\[1em] \hline \\ -\frac{(\mu+\lambda)}{4h^2}\left(\left[\begin{bmatrix}1 & 0 & -1\end{bmatrix}[0]\begin{bmatrix}-1 & 0 & 1\end{bmatrix}\right]u_1 + \left[\begin{bmatrix}1\\0\\-1\end{bmatrix}[0]\begin{bmatrix}-1\\0\\1\end{bmatrix}\right]u_2\right) \\ \quad -\left(\mu\Delta_h + \frac{\mu+\lambda}{h^2}\left[[1][-2][1]\right]\right)u_3 \end{cases}$$

For the actual computation of the solution u we employ a multi-scale approach that is wrapped around algorithm 1. There are two basic reasons to adopt such a procedure. These are reduced computational cost and robustness. The amount of data to be processed decreases with $\mathcal{O}((h'/h)^d)$, where h' is the distance between grid points on a coarser grid. Furthermore large deformations on the fine grid can be computed faster and more robustly, since they correspond to smaller deformations on coarser grids. Correspondence problems due to locally alike substructures are also avoided.

Algorithm 2 approximate a solution u^* on one grid

1: **function** APPROXSOLUTION(T, R, G, u)
2:     $k \leftarrow 0$
3:     $G_0 \leftarrow \phi_k(G_U) \cup G_V$
4:     $u_0 \leftarrow u$
5:     **repeat**
6:         calculate $f(u^{(k)}(x))$
7:         compute $d^{(k)}$
8:         $s^{(k)} \leftarrow d^{(k)}/\|d^{(k)}\|_\infty$
9:         compute τ_k by solving problem (3.3)
10:       $u^{(k+1)} \leftarrow u^{(k)} + \tau_k s^{(k)}$
11:       $k \leftarrow k+1$
12:       $G_k \leftarrow \phi_k(G_U) \cup G_V$
13:     **until** ($\|f(u^{(k)}(x))\|^2 \leq \epsilon$ or $k = k_{\max}$)
14:     $u \leftarrow u^{(k)}$
15: **end function**

The multi-scale approach is based on a Gaussian pyramid. We require that $n = 2^r + 1$, $r \in \mathbb{N}$. We define a series of grids $\{\bar{\Omega}^d_{h_l}\}_{l=\lfloor \log_2 n \rfloor, \ldots, 2, 1}$, where

$$h_l = 1/(n_l - 1) \quad \text{and} \quad n_l = 2^l + 1.$$

Then we have

$$\Omega^d_{h_i} \subset \Omega^d_{h_j} \quad \text{and} \quad \Gamma^d_{h_i} \subset \Gamma^d_{h_j}, \qquad i < j.$$

In terms of grid points $x_{i_1 \ldots i_d}$ that means

$$x_{i_1 \ldots i_d} = x'_{m(i_1 \ldots i_d)}, \quad x \in \bar{\Omega}^d_{h_j}, \; x' \in \bar{\Omega}^d_{h_k}, \; j < k, \; m = 2^{k-j}.$$

We say $\Omega^d_{h_i}$ is coarser than $\Omega^d_{h_j}$ when $i < j$, respectively finer in case $i > j$.
Using a Gaussian pyramid implies smoothing the data before sub sampling. One possible way to do this is using a binomial filter of width 3

$$\frac{1}{64} \left[\begin{bmatrix} 1 & 2 & 1 \\ 2 & 4 & 2 \\ 1 & 2 & 1 \end{bmatrix} \begin{bmatrix} 2 & 4 & 2 \\ 4 & 8 & 4 \\ 2 & 4 & 2 \end{bmatrix} \begin{bmatrix} 1 & 2 & 1 \\ 2 & 4 & 2 \\ 1 & 2 & 1 \end{bmatrix} \right]. \tag{16}$$

Note that this corresponds to the full-weighting transfer operator used in the standard multigrid. In analogy the multigrid we call the coarsening *restriction*. When transferring u to a coarser grid the boundary points need not be smoothed, since we have Dirichlet boundary conditions, $u(x) = 0 \; \forall x \in \Gamma^d_h$. That corresponds to the injection transfer operator. After computing the solution u on one grid it has to be interpolated to the next finer grid. Inverting the transfer operator described above results in trilinear interpolation.

Pseudocode algorithms for the approximation of u on each level (Algorithm 2), and the multi-scale scheme (Algorithm 3) are given. The MULTISCALE function calls itself recursively until a defined level, $\text{level}_{\text{stop}}$, is reached. Then APPROXSOLUTION performs at most $k_{\max}$ iterations on that level. On return from the recursion the solution u' from the coarser grid is interpolated to the current grid. This approximation then serves as the starting point for the iteration on that level.

For line 7 in algorithm 2 a large sparse system of linear equations has to be solved. We use a standard multigrid algorithm (with optimal multigrid complexity $\mathcal{O}(N)$ for N picture elements) as a solver, for details see e.g. [20, 18]. Yet any other solver, such as a fast discrete Fourier transformation (FFT) [28] or Krylov subspace methods [27], can be used.

5 Examples

In this section we demonstrate our algorithm on two examples. In both application the missing region will only be in the template. First we give a two dimensional example since principal effects of extending the energy functional are easier

A Mathematical Image Registration Model with Incomplete Image Information

Algorithm 3 compute solutions u on different scales starting with the coarsest on defined by level$_{stop}$

```
 1: function MULTISCALE(T, R, G, u,level)
 2:     if level=level_stop then                    ▷ stop at level_stop
 3:         approxsolution(T, R, G, u)
 4:     else
 5:         T' ← restrict(T)
 6:         R' ← restrict(R)
 7:         G' ← restrict(G)
 8:         u' ← restrict(u)
 9:         multiscale(T', R', u', G',level-1)
10:         u ← interpolate(u')
11:         approxsolution(T, R, G, u)
12:     end if
13: end function
```

to demonstrate and visualize in two dimensions. Here the input data consists of digitized histological sections of a human postmortem brain that have been stained for cell bodies. In the second example we use three dimensional volume data of the human brain. It will be demonstrated how lesions can be mapped into a reference space and an example of comparison to atlas data will be given.

In the following we use the term incomplete template for the template in which a region is missing or damaged, complete template otherwise. The region G is defined by a mask, where values greater 0 imply that the point is in G. In both examples we defined the incomplete regions ourselves. This allows for the comparison with the results of the registration with the complete templates. In most applications a complete template is not available and the missing region has to be defined by an expert.

5.1 Incomplete Histological Sections

The data in this example consists of histological sections of the human brain (256×256). With such sections the structure of the brain can be studied at a microscopical level. The sections were obtained from a human postmortem brain. With a microtome $20 \mu m$ thick sections are cut from a paraffin embedded brain. In the course of cutting, the section "wrinkle" and fold up. They have to be straightened out in a warm water bath. The deformations that are introduced in this process have to reversed when one wants to reconstruct the brain from the digitized sections. In addition to the deformations the section might tear in some regions or parts may be torn of. This is one source of problems brain volume reconstruction from sections.

We generated a template (figure 2(b)) by registering the reference (figure 2(a)) to another section. Then we "damaged" the template (figure 2(c)) by erasing a region defined by a mask (figure 2(d)). The white contour corresponds to the silouhette of the reference.

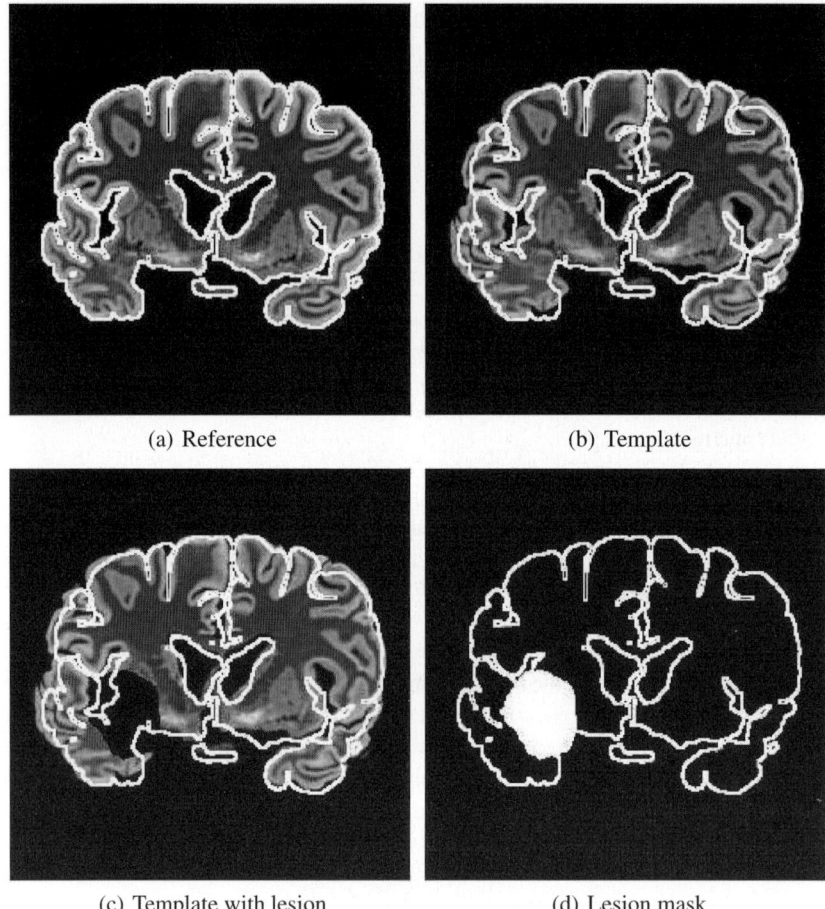

Fig. 2. Here the reference 2(a), template 2(b), template with lesion 2(c) and lesion mask 2(d) are displayed. The white contour around the sections corresponds to the silhouette of the reference.

Three different registrations were performed with identical parameters:

- registration of the complete template to the reference,
- registration of the damaged template to the reference without the extended energy functional
- registration of the damaged template to the reference with the extended energy functional.

The first one serves as a reference to which the latter two can be compared. In figures 3–5 the results for all three registrations are shown. Here in each figure, the left image (a) shows the transformed templates and in the right one the template is shown along with the deformation vector field.

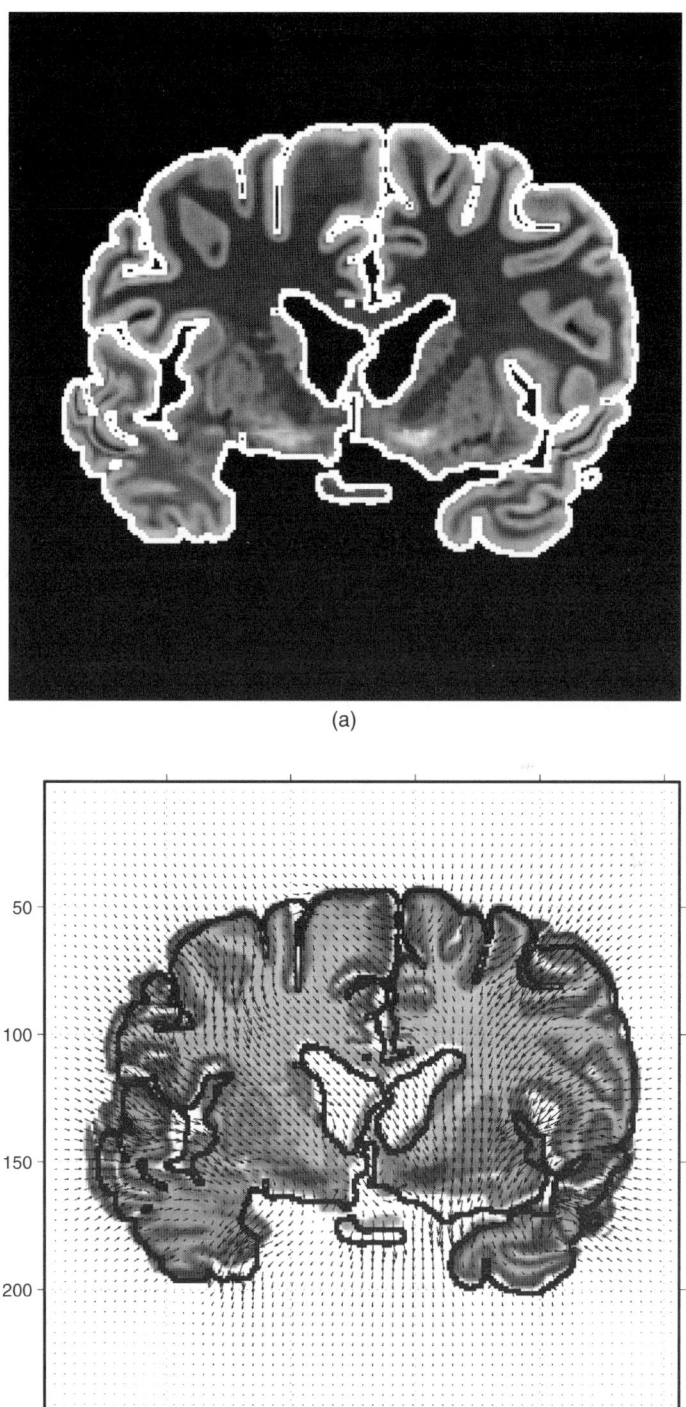

Fig. 3. Registration of the complete template. (a) shows the transformed templates. (b) the template is shown along with the deformation vector field. Both images are presented with superimposed reference contour.

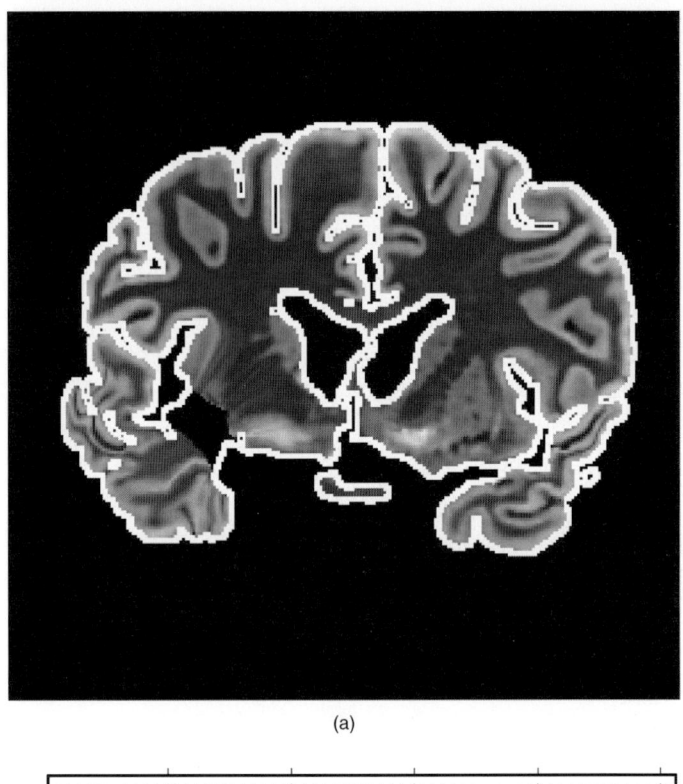

(a)

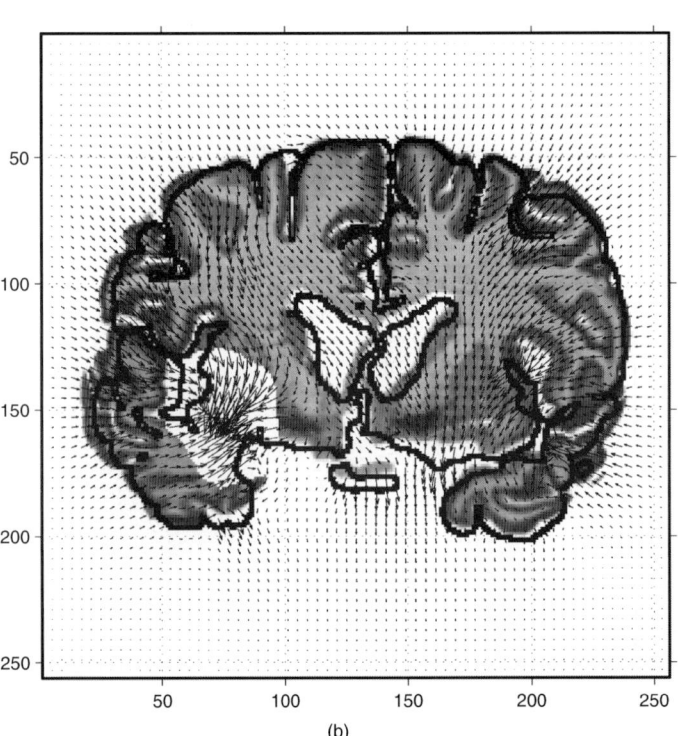

(b)

Fig. 4. Registration of the incomplete template. (a) shows the transformed templates. (b) the template is shown along with the deformation vector field. Both images are presented with superimposed reference contour.

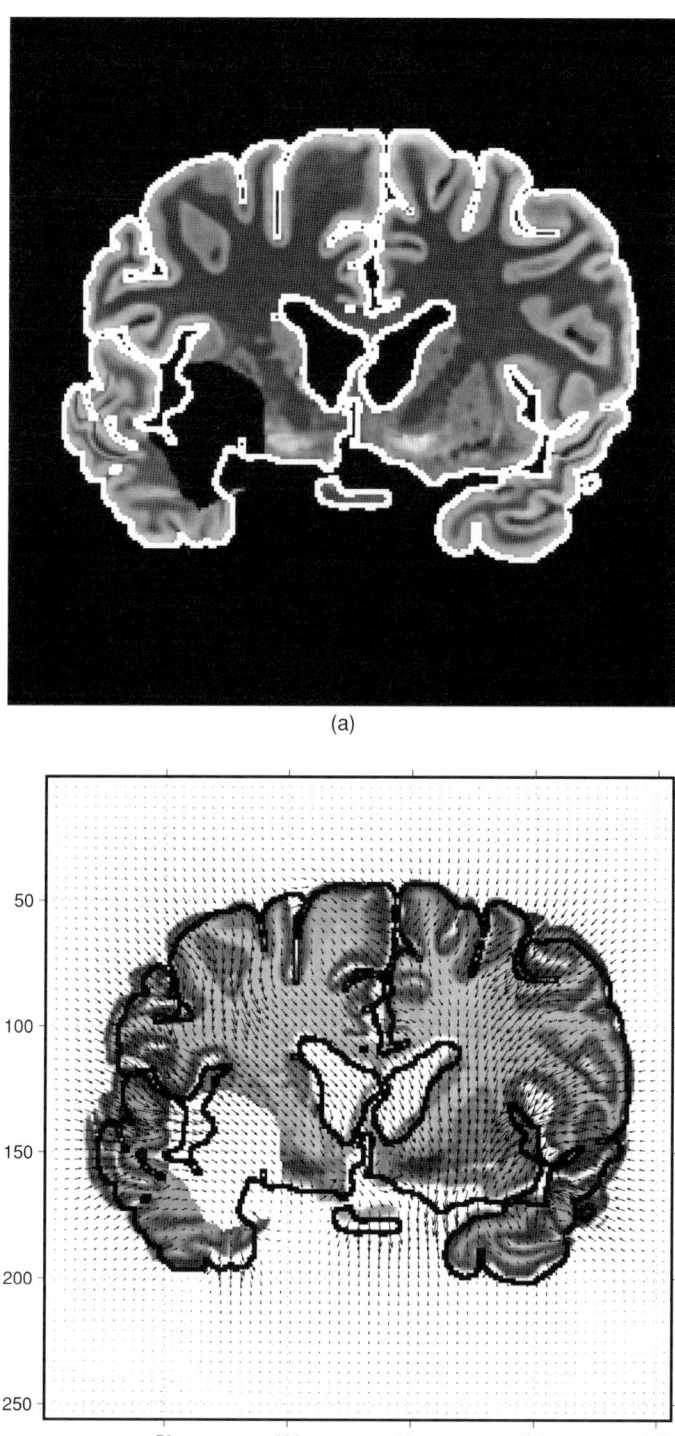

Fig. 5. Registration of the incomplete template and the additional information about the missing region. (a) shows the transformed templates. (b) the template is shown along with the deformation vector field. Both images are presented with superimposed reference contour.

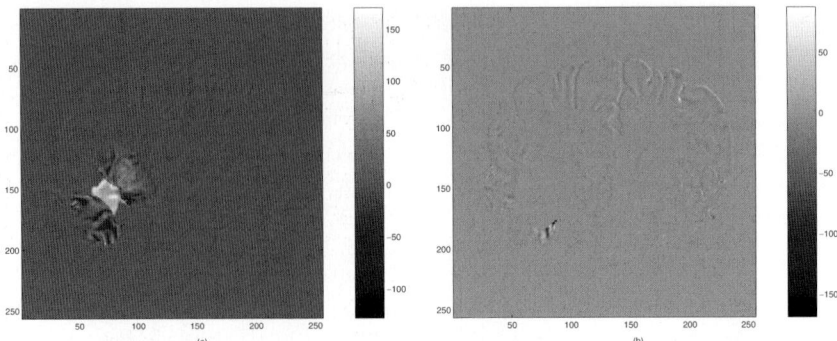

Fig. 6. Here the differences between the result of the registration with the complete template and the registrations with the incomplete template are displayed. Figure (a) shows the difference with the incomplete template without providing information about the lesion. In Figure (b) the difference with the registration with the extended energy functional is shown

It is obvious that in the second registration tissue from the surrounding area is pulled into the missing region. That is to be expected, since that minimizes the difference between template and reference. With the extended energy functional the difference in that region is not taken into account, i.e. the "force" is zero in that region. The deformation is interpolated into the missing region by the regularizing term of the equation (figure 5(b)).

The effect is visible in figure 6, too. Here the difference between the result of the registration with the complete template and the other two registrations is displayed. We chose the difference over the squared difference, since small deviations would not be visible otherwise. There are two important points to make. First, the lesion affects the transformation on the whole regardless which method is employed. That is due to the fact that a global functional is minimized, and hence the effect of local variations is propagated over the whole solution. Second, the proposed approach only works well in regions, where "sufficient information" is present in vicinity of the lesion. The only large difference with the proposed method occurs in a region where we find a small isolated structure.

5.2 Lesion Mapping

As mentioned earlier lesioned brains pose a particular problem to most registration algorithms, since the assumption about structural correspondence between reference and template is not satisfied anymore. Yet, when registering lesions to a reference atlas, it is paramount that the lesions are preserved by the registration. There have been attempts to register the lesions manually. Interactive manual mapping is prone to observer dependent bias. Additionally only simple deformation models can be used. Thus automatic, observer-independent methods that preserve the lesions are needed.

In this example we have taken a MR volume data set ($256 \times 256 \times 256$) of a healthy human male (figure ??), and segmented parts of the postcentral gyrus (figure ??). The postcentral gyrus (*gyrus postcentralis*) belongs to the sensory cortex and lies "behind" the sulcus centralis. The precentral gyrus (*gyrus precentralis*) is always in "front" of the sulcus centralis and belongs to the motor cortex. All surface renderings in figure A show top views of the brain, where the frontal part of the brain is always at the top of the image. All slices shown in this section do have the same orientation. The brain is registered to a reference brain (figure ??)[24]. The deformed lesion mask was then compared with probabilistic cytoarchiteconic maps that reside in the reference space.

These maps comprise data from 10 postmortem brains. They were constructed by registering the brains, along with the cortical region labels obtained from cytoarchitectonic studies on histological sections, to the reference brain. The degree of overlap of the labels from different brains for a certain region constitutes the probability for a voxel to belong to that region. Here we use the maps that contain the 50%-isocontours, the so called 50% maps.

Again we performed the same three registration as in the two-dimensional case above. Figure B shows the reference, the template and the results for one horizontal slice of the volume data set. The corresponding masks are overlayed in red. For the registration results the original mask has been transformed with the corresponding deformation-field. Again it is obvious that when no information about the lesion is provided the missing region is filled with surrounding tissue. As a result the lesion mask is compressed (figure ??). A comparison of figure ?? and figure ?? shows that the lesion is well preserved when a lesion mask is provided.

Figure C shows the overlayed 50% maps for Brodmann areas 1, 2, 3a, 3b, 4a, 4p [16][15][14] for the registration with the lesion mask. Sensory areas 1, 2, 3a, 3b can always be found on the gyrus postcentralis whereas motor areas 4a and 4p occupy the gyrus precentralis.

The overlayed probability maps have exactly that characteristic. Areas 4a, 4p are on the gyrus precentralis, whereas all the other areas are on the gyrus postcentralis. To quantify to which extend the regions are within the lesion we compute the voxel overlap of the maps with the transformed mask (table 1). Note that the overall voxel numbers for the maps include both hemispheres. Registration with the complete

cortical area	voxel overlap			#voxels in map
	without lesion	with mask	without mask	
1	5087	4659	1065	13340
2	49	47	0	5399
3a	2139	1997	195	11025
3b	4295	3754	475	13776
4a	418	571	138	14478
4p	536	744	73	6925

Table 1. Voxel overlap of deformed lesion mask with the probability maps for all three registrations performed.

template and incomplete template with lesion mask yield similar results. In the case where no lesion mask is provided the mask is displaced and the overlap with the maps decreases. If this would be a real patient brain, we could now correlate our findings with results from other modalities such as behavioral tests [4].

References

1. Y. Amit: A nonlinear variational problem for image matching, SIAM J. Sci. Comput **15/1**, pp 207-224, (1994)
2. R. Bajcsy and S. Kovacic: Multiresolution elastic matching, Computer Vision, **46**, pp 1-21, (1989)
3. M. Bertalmio, G. Sapiro, V. Caselles and C. Ballester: Image inpainting, Kurt Akeley (Ed), Siggraph 2000, Computer Graphics Proceedings, pp 417-424. ACM Press / ACM SIGGRAPH / Addison Wesley Longman, (2000)
4. S. Bohlhalter, C. Fretz, and B. Weder: Hierarchical versus parallel processing in tactile object recognition - a behaviouralneuroanatomical study of aperceptive tactile agnosia, Brain **125**, pp 2537-2548, (2002)
5. T. F. Chan, S. Kang and J. Shen: Euler's elastica and curvature based inpaintings, Journal on Applied Mathematics, (2002)
6. T. F. Chan and J. Shen: Mathematical models for local nontexture inpaintings, SIAM Journal on Applied Mathematics, **62/3**, pp 1019-1043, (2002)
7. G. E. Christensen, T. F. Miller, M. Vannier, and U. Grenander: Individualizing neuroanatomical atlases using a massively parallel computer, IEEE Computer, **29/1**, pp 32-38, (1996)
8. U. Clarenz, S. Henn, M. Rumpf and K. Witsch: Relations between optimization and gradient flow methods with application to image registration, Proceedings of the 18th GAMM-Seminar Leipzig, (2002)
9. E. D'Agostino, J. Modersitzki, F. Maes, D. Vandermeulen, B. Fischer and P. Suetens: Free-form registration using mutual information and curvature regularization, Preprint A-03-05, Institute of Mathematics, Medical University of Lübeck, (2003)
10. M. H. Davis, A. Khotanzad, D. Flaming and S. Harms: A physics based coordinate transformation for 3d medical images, IEEE Trans. on medical imaging, **16/3**, pp 317-328, (1997)
11. M. Droske and M. Rumpf: A variational approach to non-rigid morphological registration, SIAM Appl. Math., **64/2**, pp 668-687, (2004)
12. J. A. Fiez, H. Damasio and T. J. Grabowski: Lesion segmentation and manual warping to a reference brain: Intra- and interobserver reliability, Human Brain Mapping, **9**, pp 192-211 (2000)
13. B. Fischer and J. Modersitzki: Curvature based image registration, JMIV, **18**, pp 81-85, (2003)
14. S. Geyer, A. Ledberg, A. Schleicher, S. Kinomura, T. Schormann, U. Bürgel, T. Klingberg, J. Larsson, K. Zilles, and P. E. Roland: Two different areas within the primary motor cortex of man, Nature, **382**, pp 805-807, (1996)
15. S. Geyer, T. Schormann, H. Mohlberg and K. Zilles: Areas 3a, 3b and 1 of human primary somatosensory cortex: Ii. spatial normalization to standard anatomical space, NeuroImage, **11**, pp 617-632, (2000)

16. C. Grefkes, S. Geyer, T. Schormann, P. E. Roland and K. Zilles: Human somatosensory area 2: Observer-independent cytoarchitectonic mapping, interindividual variability and population map, NeuroImage, **14**, pp 617-632, (2001)
17. W. Hackbusch: Elliptic Differential Equations. Theory and Numerical Treatment, Springer Series in Computational Mathematics **18**, Springer-Verlag, Berlin Heidelberg New York, (1992)
18. S. Henn: Numerische Lösung und Modellierung eines inversen Problems zur Assimilation digitaler Bilddaten, Phd thesis Heinrich-Heine-Universität Düsseldorf, Logos-Verlag Berlin, Berlin Heidelberg New York, (2001)
19. S. Henn: A levenberg-marquardt scheme for nonlinear image registration, BIT Numerical Mathematics, **43/4**, pp 743-759, (2003)
20. S. Henn and K. Witsch: A multigrid-approach for minimizing a nonlinear functional for digital image matching, Computing, **64/4**, pp 339-348, (1999)
21. S. Henn and K. Witsch: Iterative multigrid regularization techniques for image matching, SIAM J. Sci. Comput. (SISC), **23/4**, pp 1077-1093, (2001)
22. S. Henn and K. Witsch: Multi-modal image registration using a variational approach, SIAM J. Sci. Comput. (SISC), **25/4**, pp 1429-1447, (2004)
23. G. Hermosillo: Variational methods for multimodal image matching, Phd thesis, Université de Nice, France, (2002)
24. C. J. Holmes, R. Hoge, L. Collins, R. Woods, A. W. Toga and A. C. Evans: Enhancement of mr images using registration for signal averaging, J. Comp. Assisted Tomogr, **22/2**, pp 324-344, (1998)
25. S. L. Keeling and W. Ring: Medical image registration and interpolation by optical flow with maximal rigidity, Journal of Mathematical Imaging and Vision JMIV, (to appear)
26. F. Maes, A. Collignon, D. Vandermeulen, G. Marchal and P. Suetens: Multimodality image registration by maximization of mutual information, IEEE transactions on Medical Imaging, **16/2**, pp 187-198, (1997)
27. Y. Saad: Iterative methods for sparse linear systems, (2000)
28. C.F. Van Loan: Computational Frameworks for the Fourier Transform, Frontiers in Applied Mathematics, **Vol. 10**, SIAM, Philadelphia, (1992)
29. W. Wells, P. Viola, H. Atsumi, S. Nakajima and R. Kikinis: Multi-modal volume registration by maximization of mutual information, Medical Image Analysis, **1**, pp 35-51, (1996)

Medical Image Registration and Interpolation by Optical Flow with Maximal Rigidity

Stephen L. Keeling

Institut für Mathematik, Karl Franzens Universität Graz
stephen.keeling@uni-graz.at

Abstract In this paper a variational method for registering or mapping like points in medical images is proposed and analyzed. The proposed variational principle penalizes a departure from rigidity and thereby provides a natural generalization of strictly rigid registration techniques used widely in medical contexts. Difficulties with finite displacements are elucidated, and alternative infinitesimal displacements are developed for an optical flow formulation which also permits image interpolation. The variational penalty against non-rigid flows provides sufficient regularization for a well-posed minimization and yet does not rule out irregular registrations corresponding to an object excision. Image similarity is measured by penalizing the variation of a local image feature along optical flow trajectories. The approach proposed here is also independent of the order in which images are taken. For computations, a lumped finite element Eulerian discretization is used to solve for the optical flow. Also, a Lagrangian integration of the intensity along optical flow trajectories has the advantage of prohibiting diffusion among trajectories which would otherwise blur interpolated images. The subtle aspects of the methods developed are illustrated in terms of simple examples, and the approach is finally applied to the registration of magnetic resonance images.

1 Introduction

The diagnostic use of medical image sets in a clinical setting implicitly requires a point by point correspondence between the same tissue sites in separate images. For example, two given images may be of a single patient at different times, such as during a mammography examination involving repeated imaging after the injection of a contrast agent [30]. On the other hand, the images may be of a single patient viewed by different imaging modalities, such as by magnetic resonance and computerized tomography to provide complementary information for image-guided surgery [13]. In fact, images of two separate patients may even be compared to evaluate the extent of pathology of one in relation to the other [34]. Similarly, an image of a patient may be compared to an idealized atlas in order to identify or segment tissue classes based upon a detailed segmentation of the atlas [34]. Thus, what is needed finally is an explicit coordinate transformation that will map any point in one image to its corresponding point in the other. With such a mapping, images are said to be *registered*.

Since the term registration is often used rather loosely in the context of its applications, it may be useful to elaborate on the above description of what registration is by stating what it is not. Note that by manipulating intensities alone, it is possible to warp or morph one image to another without having an explicit coordinate transformation identifying like image points. Thus image registration is not image morphing, but can be used for such an application. Similarly, image interpolation can be achieved without registration, but a parameterized coordinate transformation can be used to interpolate between images. Also, when complementary information in separate imaging modalities is superimposed, images are said to be *fused*. Since fusion too can be achieved by manipulating intensities alone, fused images need not be registered, but rather *can* be fused by registration.

Rigid registration is performed under the constraint that images are related by a pure rigid-body transformation, i.e., a translation plus a rotation. Such registration is attractive in medical imaging because of the ubiquity of nearly rigid objects in the body. It is especially popular for image modality fusion in order to guide brain surgery [13]. Particularly when performed prospectively with the use of extrinsic fiducial markers, rigid registration and its concomitant errors are well understood [14]. Since rigid registration is widely used and treated as a standard for comparison in the medical community [13], even in cases for which a more flexible registration is sought [30], it was an initial aim of the present work to define a generalization which maximizes rigidity in a natural sense.

A leading application and demand for non-rigid registration is for mammographic image sequences in which tissue deformations are less rigid and more elastic [30]. This observation has motivated the development of registration methods based on linear elasticity [12], [28], but difficulties resulting from finite displacements will be elucidated here. Alternatives emerge from noting that a rigid transformation is equivalent to one which is both conformal (angle preserving) and isometric (area preserving) [7]. Some authors relax rigidity by constraining transformations to be conformal or isometric [15]. Others employ a local rigidity constraint [21] or allow identified objects to move as rigid bodies [22]. The approach developed here involves instead a variational principle penalizing a departure from rigidity. Thus, a rigid registration is selected when one fits the data. Otherwise rigidity is maximized strongly or weakly depending upon the dominance of the rigidity penalty. Based upon a function space minimization, this approach is non-parametric. By contrast, many other non-rigid registration methods are parametric, based for instance upon the determination of polynomial coefficients [30].

Whether parametric or non-parametric, the unknowns in a registration problem are generally over-determined by the available information, and must be determined by optimizing an image similarity measure; see [13] for further details. When two images are related by a simple misalignment, the sum of squared intensity differences is a natural similarity measure. Statistical measures have also been employed, and the correlation coefficient has been recognized as ideal when the intensities of the two images are related by a linear rescaling [37]. Also, the adaptation of thermodynamic entropy for information theory has suggested mutual information as an image similarity measure [24] [40], and a heuristically based normalized mutual information has been found to work very well in practice [31]. While simple examples can be constructed to demonstrate the advantages and disadvantages of these measures in relation to each other, it is a noteworthy conclusion of the study in [41] that highly accurate rigid registrations of multi-modal brain images can be achieved with information-theoretic measures. Nevertheless, as recognized in [29], mutual information contains no local spatial information, and random pixel perturbations leave underlying entropies unchanged. Higher order entropies including probabilities of neighboring pixel pairs can be employed to achieve superior results for non-rigid registration [29]; however, the message is that local spatial information in an image similarity measure is advantageous. Thus, in the present framework image similarity is driven by penalizing the variation of a local image feature along trajectores connecting like points. In the present work, the investigated local image feature is the scaled intensity, but other discussed features can be treated naturally.

Without regularization the ill-posed process of image registration can lead to quite aberrant results, particularly when it is performed parametrically and especially when it is performed under landmark constraints [25]. Specifically, a landmark constraint is a required correspondence between points generally identified retrospectively and either automatically or manually [28]. Parametric spline-based formulations in particular are readily amenable to regularization for instance by penalizing second order derivatives [30]. Such curvature based regularization has also been applied non-parametrically [11]. In the approach developed here, a variational penalty on the departure from rigidity provides sufficient regularization for a well-posed minimization. At the same time, the penalty does not rule out irregular registrations, for example, corresponding to an object excision.

The approach developed in this work was influenced by Thirion's interpretation of optical flow as a means of driving a diffusion process in which one image is deformed toward a match with a static second image [33]. This process may be visualized in Fig. 1 with the deformations evolving from the front face (shown right) toward the back face (shown left) of the displayed box. Because of an apparent unnatural directionality in this diffusion process, the present work was oriented from the outset so that the registration would be the same independent of the order in which images are taken; see also [5]. With this preconception, one might already anticipate an elliptic formulation in the box of Fig. 1, with the given images imposed as boundary conditions on the front and back faces. In fact, an elliptic system is derived here for an optical flow field whose integrated trajectories connect like image points in the front and back faces. Natural boundary conditions also permit trajectories to leave the computational domain, which is a necessary condition to support purely rigid transformations. Furthermore, image interpolation is achieved in parallel image planes by distributing the (optimally scaled) intensity with minimal variation along trajectories. Thus, while the optical flow is determined in an Eulerian frame, the intensity is determined in a Lagrangian frame, which has the advantage of prohibiting diffusion among trajectories which would otherwise blur interpolated images. Note that optical flow has been proposed in other ways for registration, but with an evolution equation formulation that depends upon the order of the images [2], and with more usual optical flow regularization that leads to aqueous effects which are unnatural for medical applications [17].

The paper can now be summarized as follows. In Section 2 a framework used throughout the paper is presented. Specifically, optical flow is defined and image similarity is developed in terms of the variation of a local image feature, such as scaled intensity, along optical flow trajectories. In Section 3 basic elements from elasticity theory are explored for registration regularization. It is shown that linearized elastic potential energy of finite displacements does not select rigid transformations preferentially, and that the unlinearized energy is computationally intractable. Finally, a computationally convenient penalty on the departure of infinitesimal displacements from rigidity is identified. Section 4 begins with a complete definition of the proposed variational registration method. Then the optimality conditions are derived separately for each variable in subsections. Simple examples are also considered to justify the choice of penalty functions and of boundary conditions. Also, the optical flow system is shown to be well-posed under the condition that the intensity does not manifest certain trivial symmetries. For the case of landmark constraints, Lagrange Multipliers are shown to exist and satisfy stationarity conditions. Section 5 begins by introducing the numerical framework for the proposed registration method. Then the discretizations of the optimality system of the previous section are developed separately for each variable in subsections. In Section 6 the final numerical implementation is applied both to test cases and to magnetic resonance images. In particular it is shown that the approach succeeds in achieving a natural generalization of rigid registration.

2 Image Similarity

Following the illustration in Fig. 1 for 2D images, let two given images I_0 and I_1 be situated respectively on the front and back faces of a box,

$$Q = \{(x_1, \ldots, x_N, z) = (\boldsymbol{x}, z) : 0 < x_1, \ldots, x_N, z < 1\}, \tag{1}$$

i.e.,

$$I_0 \text{ on } \Omega_0 = \{(\boldsymbol{x}, z) \in \partial Q : z = 0\} \tag{2}$$

and

$$I_1 \text{ on } \Omega_1 = \{(\boldsymbol{x}, z) \in \partial Q : z = 1\}. \tag{3}$$

Then define curvilinear coordinates $(\xi_1, \ldots, \xi_N, \zeta) = (\boldsymbol{\xi}, \zeta)$ so that $\boldsymbol{\xi}$ is constant along trajectories through Q that connect like points in I_0 and I_1, and $\zeta = z$. Also, suppose that $\boldsymbol{x} = \boldsymbol{\xi}$ in Ω_0 and therefore the displacement vector within Q is $\boldsymbol{d} = \boldsymbol{x} - \boldsymbol{\xi}$. Further, a trajectory tangent is given by $(u_1, \ldots, u_N, 1)$ in terms of the optical flow defined as

$$\boldsymbol{u} = (u_1, \ldots, u_N) = \boldsymbol{x}_\zeta. \tag{4}$$

Now the simplest similarity measure described in Section 1, i.e., the sum of squared intensity differences, takes the following form,

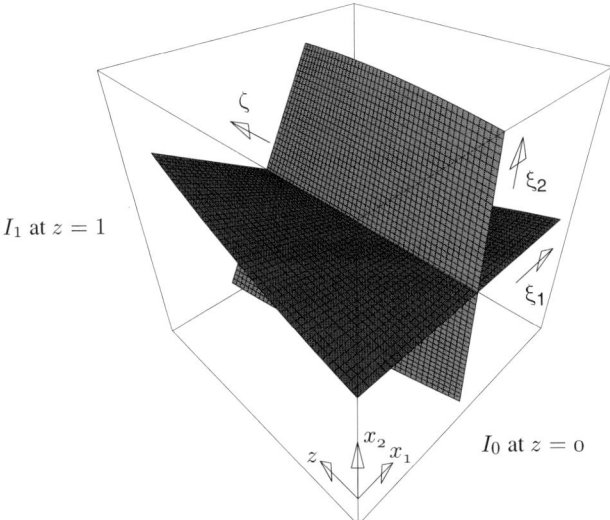

Fig. 1. The domain Q with 2D images I_0 and I_1 on the front and back faces Ω_0 and Ω_1, respectively. Curvilinear coordinates are defined to be constant on trajectories connecting like points in I_0 and I_1.

$$\int_{\Omega_0^c} [I_0(\boldsymbol{\xi}) - I_1(\boldsymbol{x}(\boldsymbol{\xi}, 1))]^2 \, d\boldsymbol{\xi}. \tag{5}$$

It is not assumed that every point in Ω_0 finds a like point in Ω_1, i.e., trajectories are allowed to move out of the box Q. Therefore, the domain of integration in (5) is given by $\Omega_0^c = \{\boldsymbol{\xi} \in \Omega_0 : \boldsymbol{x}(\boldsymbol{\xi}, \zeta) \in Q, 0 < \zeta < 1\}$, the subset of Ω_0 on which trajectories extend completely through the full depth of Q. To reach a similarity measure which involves only infinitesimal displacements as opposed to the finite displacement $\boldsymbol{d}(\boldsymbol{\xi}, 1) = \boldsymbol{x}(\boldsymbol{\xi}, 1) - \boldsymbol{\xi}$, consider now the integral,

$$\int_0^1 \int_{\Omega_0^c} \left[\frac{dI}{d\zeta}(\boldsymbol{x}(\boldsymbol{\xi}, \zeta), \zeta) \right]^2 d\boldsymbol{\xi} d\zeta, \tag{6}$$

constrained by the boundary conditions:

$$I(\boldsymbol{\xi}, 0) = I_0(\boldsymbol{\xi}), \quad I(\boldsymbol{x}(\boldsymbol{\xi}, 1), 1) = I_1(\boldsymbol{x}(\boldsymbol{\xi}, 1)), \quad \boldsymbol{\xi} \in \Omega_0^c. \tag{7}$$

To demonstrate the relation between (5) and (6), consider that, under the condition (7), (6) is minimized by:

$$I(\boldsymbol{x}(\boldsymbol{\xi}, \zeta), \zeta) = I_0(\boldsymbol{\xi}) + \zeta[I_1(\boldsymbol{x}(\boldsymbol{\xi}, 1)) - I_0(\boldsymbol{\xi})]. \tag{8}$$

Substituting this expression into (6) then leads back to (5). However, with (4) the optical flow equation [18]:

$$\frac{dI}{d\zeta}(\boldsymbol{x}(\boldsymbol{\xi},\zeta),\zeta) = \nabla_{\boldsymbol{x}} I \cdot \boldsymbol{x}_\zeta + I_\zeta = \nabla_{\boldsymbol{x}} I \cdot \boldsymbol{u} + I_z, \qquad (9)$$

now suggests the following modification of (6),

$$\int_Q [\nabla_{\boldsymbol{x}} I \cdot \boldsymbol{u} + I_z]^2 \, d\boldsymbol{x} dz, \qquad (10)$$

which has an integrand involving purely local information throughout Q. It differs from (6) by not including the transformation Jacobian $1/\det(\nabla_\xi \boldsymbol{x})$. In other words, (10) gives a convenient *Eulerian* (local) counterpart to the *Lagrangian* (trajectory following) form appearing in (6). Furthermore, the counterpart to (7) in the Eulerian context is given by:

$$I = I_0 \text{ on } \Omega_0, \qquad I = I_1 \text{ on } \Omega_1. \qquad (11)$$

It is also shown by a consideration of optimality conditions in Section 4 that a minimizer I for (10) should satisfy the supplementary boundary condition:

$$I = 0 \text{ on } \Gamma = \partial Q \setminus \{\Omega_0 \cup \Omega_1\}. \qquad (12)$$

Thus, an image similarity measure is given by (10) under the constraints (11) and (12).

Other similarity measures can be treated along the same lines. Specifically, suppose $\mathcal{D}$ is an operator which extracts a local image feature which should differ as little as possible between like points in the images I_0 and I_1. Then subject to the new boundary conditions,

$$I = \mathcal{D} I_0 \text{ on } \Omega_0, \qquad I = \mathcal{D} I_1 \text{ on } \Omega_1, \qquad (13)$$

the function I in (10) transports the chosen feature along optical flow trajectores. For instance, $\mathcal{D}$ may be a differential operator designed to match level curves. Of course, other differential geometric or statistical descriptors can be treated naturally. In particular, intensity scaling is considered here.

Specifically, suppose $\boldsymbol{x}^*(\boldsymbol{\xi},1)$ is an error-free registration. As explained in Section 1, because of acquisition differences, the intensity function $I_0(\boldsymbol{\xi})$ can possess a different scaling in relation to $I_1(\boldsymbol{x}^*(\boldsymbol{\xi},1))$. In other words, there may exist a function $\sigma^*(\iota)$ such that $\sigma^*(I_0(\boldsymbol{\xi})) = I_1(\boldsymbol{x}^*(\boldsymbol{\xi},1))$. However, since the number of quantized intensity values may be quite different in the two images I_0 and I_1, a reciprocal formulation requires that both images be scaled; see Subsection 4.2. Thus, unknown scaling functions $\sigma_0(\iota)$ and $\sigma_1(\iota)$ are introduced in (5) through the new residual $[\sigma_0(I_0(\boldsymbol{\xi})) - \sigma_1(I_1(\boldsymbol{x}(\boldsymbol{\xi},1)))]^2$. Similarly, σ_0 and σ_1 are introduced into (10) through the boundary conditions:

$$I = \sigma_0(I_0) \text{ on } \Omega_0, \qquad I = \sigma_1(I_1) \text{ on } \Omega_1. \qquad (14)$$

Thus, an image similarity measure incorporating scaling functions is given by (10) under the constraints (12) and (14).

3 Elastic Regularization

For a given ζ in Fig. 1, consider now the deformation $x(\xi, \zeta)$ and the associated matrix (the right Cauchy-Green strain tensor in elasticity [7]),

$$C(\zeta) = \nabla_\xi x^T \nabla_\xi x = \{\nabla_\xi x_i \cdot \nabla_\xi x_j\}. \tag{1}$$

The transformation is conformal if $\nabla_\xi x_i \cdot \nabla_\xi x_j = 0$, $i \neq j$, and additionally isometric if $\|\nabla_\xi x_i\|^2 = 1$, $i = 1, \ldots, N$, and so rigid when $C(\zeta) = I$ [7]. Thus, the (Green-St.Venant) strain $E = \frac{1}{2}(C - I)$ measures how close the deformation is to being rigid. The work required to perform a given deformation gives the elastic potential energy stored in the deformed body [7],

$$W(E) = \int_{\Omega_0^c} \left[\lambda \operatorname{tr}(E)^2 + 2\mu |E|^2 \right] d\xi, \tag{2}$$

where λ and μ are the so-called Lamé constants [7]. Here, $|E|^2 = E : E$ where : denotes a componentwise matrix scalar product. Now in terms of the displacement $d = x - \xi$ the strain can be linearized according to $2E = C - I = \nabla_\xi d + \nabla_\xi d^T + \nabla_\xi d^T \nabla_\xi d \approx \nabla_\xi d + \nabla_\xi d^T$ which gives the approximation to the elastic potential energy,

$$W(E) \approx \int_{\Omega_0^c} \left[\lambda (\nabla_\xi \cdot d)^2 + \tfrac{1}{2}\mu \left| \nabla_\xi d^T + \nabla_\xi d \right|^2 \right] d\xi. \tag{3}$$

With (5) and (3), consider (tentatively) computing a registration by minimizing the following cost,

$$J_{\text{lin}}(d) = \int_{\Omega_0^c} [I_0(\xi) - I_1(\xi + d(\xi, 1))]^2 \, d\xi$$

$$+ \int_0^1 \int_{\Omega_0^c} \left[\lambda (\nabla_\xi \cdot d)^2 + \frac{\mu}{2} \left| \nabla_\xi d^T + \nabla_\xi d \right|^2 + \nu (d_\zeta \cdot d_{\zeta\zeta})^2 \right] d\xi \, d\zeta \tag{4}$$

where the term $\nu(d_\zeta \cdot d_{\zeta\zeta})^2$ is included for regularity in the depth direction and also to vanish for a natural rigid transformation. The following reasoning shows that (3) is not a suitable regularization for selecting rigid transformations. Suppose I_0 and I_1 are related by a rigid transformation r via $I_0(\xi) = I_1(r(\xi))$. Clearly the choice of a morphing $x(\xi, \zeta)$ in which r can be embedded via $x(\xi, 0) = \xi$ and $x(\xi, 1) = r(\xi)$ is not unique. Specifically, define the rigid-body motion,

$$\hat{x}(\xi, \zeta) = R(\zeta)(\xi - a) + a, \tag{5}$$

where a is the center of rotation and $R(\zeta) = e^{\zeta W}$ for a skew-symmetrix matrix W [26]. Also define the convex combination $\tilde{x}(\xi, \zeta) = (1-\zeta)\xi + \zeta \hat{x}(\xi, 1)$, which with increasing ζ corresponds to compressing the initial image and then expanding it to the final image. Assume further that the intensities corresponding to these transformations are given in Q by (8) with x replaced by $\hat{x}$ and $\tilde{x}$ respectively. With this choice, the similarity term (5) is zero. Now, with $\hat{\boldsymbol{d}} = \hat{\boldsymbol{x}} - \boldsymbol{\xi}$ and $\tilde{\boldsymbol{d}} = \tilde{\boldsymbol{x}} - \boldsymbol{\xi}$, an elementary calculation shows that $J_{\text{lin}}(\tilde{\boldsymbol{d}}) < J_{\text{lin}}(\hat{\boldsymbol{d}})$. In other words, the linearized elastic potential energy regularization selects the compression/expansion instead of the rigid-body motion.

The situation is different for the unlinearized elastic potential energy. Using (5) and (2) to define the cost,

$$J_{\text{unl}}(\boldsymbol{x}) = \int_{\Omega_0^c} [I_0(\boldsymbol{\xi}) - I_1(\boldsymbol{x}(\boldsymbol{\xi}, 1))]^2 \, d\boldsymbol{\xi}$$

$$+ \frac{\lambda}{4} \int_0^1 \int_{\Omega_0^c} \left[\sum_{i=1}^N (\|\nabla_{\boldsymbol{\xi}} x_i\|^2 - 1) \right]^2 d\boldsymbol{\xi} d\zeta$$

$$+ \frac{\mu}{2} \int_0^1 \int_{\Omega_0^c} \left[\sum_{i=1}^N (\|\nabla_{\boldsymbol{\xi}} x_i\|^2 - 1)^2 + \sum_{i \neq j} (\nabla_{\boldsymbol{\xi}} x_i \cdot \nabla_{\boldsymbol{\xi}} x_j)^2 \right] d\boldsymbol{\xi} d\zeta \quad (6)$$

$$+ \nu \int_0^1 \int_{\Omega_0^c} (\boldsymbol{x}_{\zeta\zeta} \cdot \boldsymbol{x}_{\zeta\zeta\zeta})^2 \, d\boldsymbol{\xi} d\zeta.$$

leads to $J_{\text{unl}}(\hat{\boldsymbol{x}}) = 0 < J_{\text{unl}}(\tilde{\boldsymbol{x}})$, and thus the unlinearized elastic potential energy regularization selects the rigid-body motion instead of the compression/expansion. However, the optimality system for J_{unl} is very complex and contains coefficients with terms $(\|\nabla_{\boldsymbol{\xi}} x_i\|^2 - 1)$ whose signs may not even be uniform.

Nevertheless, these difficulties can be circumvented by formulating rigidity in an Eulerian frame instead of in a Lagrangian frame. To this end, note that $\boldsymbol{x}_\zeta(\boldsymbol{\xi}, \zeta) = \boldsymbol{u}(\boldsymbol{x}(\boldsymbol{\xi}, \zeta), \zeta)$ gives $\nabla_{\boldsymbol{\xi}} \boldsymbol{x}_\zeta = \nabla_{\boldsymbol{x}} \boldsymbol{u} \nabla_{\boldsymbol{\xi}} \boldsymbol{x}$, and therefore $C(\zeta)$ in (1) satisfies:

$$\partial_\zeta C(\zeta) = \nabla_{\boldsymbol{\xi}} \boldsymbol{x}_\zeta^T \nabla_{\boldsymbol{\xi}} \boldsymbol{x} + \nabla_{\boldsymbol{\xi}} \boldsymbol{x}^T \nabla_{\boldsymbol{\xi}} \boldsymbol{x}_\zeta = \nabla_{\boldsymbol{\xi}} \boldsymbol{x}^T \left[\nabla_{\boldsymbol{x}} \boldsymbol{u}^T + \nabla_{\boldsymbol{x}} \boldsymbol{u} \right] \nabla_{\boldsymbol{\xi}} \boldsymbol{x}. \quad (7)$$

Hence, if $\nabla_{\boldsymbol{x}} \boldsymbol{u}$ is skew-symmetric, then $\partial_\zeta C(\zeta) = 0$ implies $C(\zeta) = C(0) = I$ and the transformation is rigid for all $\zeta \in [0, 1]$.

Now with (10) and (7), consider computing a registration by minimizing the following cost,

$$J_{\text{eul}}(I, \boldsymbol{u}) = \int_Q \left[(\nabla_{\boldsymbol{x}} I \cdot \boldsymbol{u} + I_z)^2 + \beta \left| \nabla_{\boldsymbol{x}} \boldsymbol{u}^T + \nabla_{\boldsymbol{x}} \boldsymbol{u} \right|^2 + \alpha |\boldsymbol{u}_z|^2 \right] d\boldsymbol{x} dz \quad (8)$$

subject to $I = I_0$ on Ω_0, $I = I_1$ on Ω_1, and $I = 0$ on Γ. The term involving $\boldsymbol{u}_z$ is included on the same grounds that ζ-derivative terms are included in (4) and (6). To test this formulation with $\hat{\boldsymbol{x}}$ and $\tilde{\boldsymbol{x}}$ as considered above, define

$$\hat{\boldsymbol{u}}(\boldsymbol{x}, z) = \hat{\boldsymbol{x}}_\zeta = W(\boldsymbol{x} - \boldsymbol{a}) \quad (9)$$

and $\tilde{u}(x, z) = \tilde{x}_\zeta = [z + (R(1) - I)^{-1}]^{-1}(x - a)$. As before, assume that the similarity term (10) is zero, which is the case for the following intensity:

$$\hat{I}(x, z) = I_0\left(R(z)^{\mathrm{T}}(x - a) + a\right). \tag{10}$$

Then an elementary calculation shows that $J_{\mathrm{eul}}(\hat{I}, \hat{u}) = 0 < J_{\mathrm{eul}}(\hat{I}, \tilde{u})$. In other words, the rigid-body motion is selected instead of the compression/expansion. It is also seen in the next section that the optimality system corresponding to (8) is computationally convenient.

Notice that (5) and (9) give the unique rigid transformation whose center of rotation is fixed globally with respect to ζ or z. Now suppose it is desired to allow some local variation in the center of rotation with respect to the depth direction. To accommodate the wider class of rigid transformations,

$$x(\xi, \zeta) = R(\zeta)(\xi - a) + (a + b\zeta), \qquad u(x, z) = W(x - a - bz) + b \tag{11}$$

in which the center of rotation $(a + bz)$ is shifted in a natural linear fashion, the cost must be modified as follows for well-posed minimization:

$$J_{\mathrm{loc}}(I, u) = \int_Q [(\nabla_x I \cdot u + I_z)^2 + \gamma \left|\nabla_x u^{\mathrm{T}} + \nabla_x u\right|^2 \\ + \beta |\nabla_x u_z|^2 + \alpha |u_{zz}|^2] dx dz. \tag{12}$$

At the other extreme is the apparently narrower class of rigid transformations which are autonomous, for which the cost may be defined as follows:

$$J_{\mathrm{aut}}(I, u) = \int_Q (\nabla_x I \cdot u + I_z)^2 \, dx dz + \int_\Omega \beta \left|\nabla_x u^{\mathrm{T}} + \nabla_x u\right|^2 dx. \tag{13}$$

The consistent trend toward autonomy among the experiments in Section 6 raises the question about when autonomous flows are selected by costs other than (13). This matter can be at least partly illuminated by demonstrating the existence of a registration which cannot be realized by an autonomous flow. For this, define the flow:

$$x_1(\xi_1, \xi_2, \zeta) = \xi_1 \cos[(\pi + \varepsilon\xi_2^2)\zeta] + \xi_2 \sin[(\pi + \varepsilon\xi_2^2)\zeta]$$
$$x_2(\xi_1, \xi_2, \zeta) = -\xi_1 \sin[(\pi + \varepsilon\xi_2^2)\zeta] + \xi_2 \cos[(\pi + \varepsilon\xi_2^2)\zeta]$$

and the discrete map $X(\xi) = x(\xi, 1)$. Note that for a given ζ and for $\varepsilon > 0$ sufficiently small, $\det(\partial x/\partial \xi) = 1 - 2\varepsilon\xi_1\xi_2\zeta > 0$ holds, and the mapping is diffeomorphic. Note also that origin centered circles are mapped onto themselves, $\|x(\xi, \zeta)\|_2 = \|\xi\|_2$, and in fact $X(\xi)$ maps the ξ_1-axis onto itself while $[X \circ X](\xi)$ is periodic on the ξ_1-axis. Given these mappings, let I_0 and I_1 be any two images which satisfy $I_0(\xi) = I_1(X(\xi))$ and which can be registered essentially only by X; e.g., suppose I_1 has uniformly distributed random intensity values. Now suppose that $\bar{u} = \bar{x}_\zeta$ is an autonomous flow field which realizes the given registration according to $\bar{x}(\xi, 1) = X(\xi)$. Then a contradiction is reached as follows; see [4].

From the phase space property, $\bar{x}(\boldsymbol{\xi}, \zeta) = \bar{x}(\bar{x}(\boldsymbol{\xi}, \tau), \zeta) = \bar{x}(\boldsymbol{\xi}, \tau + \zeta) = \bar{x}(\bar{x}(\boldsymbol{\xi}, \zeta), \tau)$, of τ-periodic autonomous flows, $\bar{x}(\boldsymbol{\xi}, 0) = \boldsymbol{\xi} = \bar{x}(\boldsymbol{\xi}, \tau)$, it follows that if $\bar{x}$ is τ-periodic at any point on a given circle, then $\bar{x}$ is τ-periodic at all points on that circle. While $\bar{x}(\boldsymbol{\xi}, 2) = \bar{x}(\bar{x}(\boldsymbol{\xi}, 1), 1) = [\boldsymbol{X} \circ \boldsymbol{X}](\boldsymbol{\xi}) = \boldsymbol{\xi}$ holds for all points $\boldsymbol{\xi}$ with $\xi_2 = 0$, it holds for no points with $\xi_2 \neq 0$, and therefore $\bar{u}$ cannot be autonomous. Further details of autonomous registrations given by (13) will be considered in detail along with (12) and with elasticity [12] and curvature [11] based regularization in forthcoming work.

4 Optimality Conditions

On the basis of previous sections, image registration and interpolation are now achieved by minimizing the following cost,

$$J(I, \sigma_0, \sigma_1, \boldsymbol{u}) = \int_Q \left[(\nabla I \cdot \boldsymbol{u} + I_z)^2 + \phi\left(|\nabla \boldsymbol{u}^T + \nabla \boldsymbol{u}|^2\right) + \alpha |\boldsymbol{u}_z|^2 \right] d\boldsymbol{x} dz \quad (1)$$

subject to:

$$I = \sigma_0(I_0) \text{ on } \Omega_0, \qquad I = \sigma_1(I_1) \text{ on } \Omega_1, \qquad \text{and} \qquad I = 0 \text{ on } \Gamma \quad (2)$$

and to possible landmark constraints:

$$x(\boldsymbol{\xi}_j, 1) = x_j, \qquad j = 1, \ldots, \hat{j} \quad (3)$$

where trajectories through the domain Q are defined by integrating the optical flow under boundary conditions, i.e., by solving:

$$\boldsymbol{x}(\boldsymbol{\xi}, \zeta) = \boldsymbol{\xi} + \int_0^\zeta \boldsymbol{u}(\boldsymbol{x}(\boldsymbol{\xi}, \rho), \rho) d\rho, \qquad \boldsymbol{\xi} \in \Omega_0, \quad \zeta \in [0, 1] \quad (4)$$

and

$$\boldsymbol{y}(\boldsymbol{\eta}, \zeta) = \boldsymbol{\eta} + \int_\zeta^1 \boldsymbol{u}(\boldsymbol{y}(\boldsymbol{\eta}, \rho), \rho) d\rho, \qquad \boldsymbol{\eta} \in \Omega_1, \quad \zeta \in [0, 1]. \quad (5)$$

A registration is given by the coordinate transformation $\boldsymbol{x}(\boldsymbol{\xi}, 1)$ and by the inverse transformation $\boldsymbol{y}(\boldsymbol{\eta}, 0)$. The given images I_0 and I_1 are interpolated by the intensity I.

The function ϕ appearing in (1) is discussed further in Subsection 4.3, but it is assumed to be smooth on $(0, \infty)$ and continuous on $[0, \infty)$. Also, the term involving $\boldsymbol{u}_z$ is included to select the most natural rigid-body motion in Q as well as to establish the well-posedness shown below in Theorem 2.

With respect to the registration goal as stated in the Introduction, it may be observed now that the formulation in Q increases the problem dimension by one. In this connection, the following points are worthwhile to emphasize. First, the present formulation affords image interpolation in addition to registration. Also, alternative diffusion processes evolving from Ω_0 to Ω_1 are here replaced by an elliptic formulation in Q with the payoff that the result is independent of the image order. Finally, these benefits are gained without an increased problem dimension if the optical flow is autonomous. Although the condition $\boldsymbol{u}_z = 0$ is not imposed explicitly in this work, it was found to hold practically in all examples presented in Section 6.

The necessary optimality conditions are now derived separately for each variable in the following subsections. The intent is to solve cyclically for one variable with the other held fixed.

4.1 Optimality Conditions for Intensity

First, for fixed σ_0, σ_1, and $\boldsymbol{u}$, the variational derivative of J with respect to I is given by:

$$\frac{\delta J}{\delta I}(I; \bar{I}) = 2 \int_Q (\boldsymbol{\nabla} I \cdot \boldsymbol{w}) \left(\boldsymbol{\nabla} \bar{I} \cdot \boldsymbol{w} \right) d\boldsymbol{y} \tag{6}$$

where for convenience $\boldsymbol{\nabla} = (\nabla, \partial_z)$, $\boldsymbol{w} = (\boldsymbol{u}, 1)$, and $\boldsymbol{y} = (\boldsymbol{x}, z)$. Also, assume for the moment that I is only subject to $I = \sigma_0(I_0)$ on Ω_0 and $I = \sigma_1(I_1)$ on Ω_1, so that the perturbation $\bar{I}$ is constrained to vanish on Ω_0 and on Ω_1. Then, boundary integrals on Ω_0 and on Ω_1 vanish in the following:

$$\begin{aligned}\frac{\delta J}{\delta I}(I; \bar{I}) &= 2 \int_{\partial Q} (\boldsymbol{\nabla} I \cdot \boldsymbol{w})(\boldsymbol{w} \cdot \boldsymbol{\nu}) \bar{I} d\boldsymbol{y} - 2 \int_Q \boldsymbol{\nabla} \cdot [(\boldsymbol{\nabla} I \cdot \boldsymbol{w}) \boldsymbol{w}] \bar{I} d\boldsymbol{y} \\ &= 2 \int_\Gamma (\boldsymbol{\nabla} I \cdot \boldsymbol{w})(\boldsymbol{u} \cdot \boldsymbol{n}) \bar{I} d\boldsymbol{y} - 2 \int_Q \boldsymbol{\nabla} \cdot [(\boldsymbol{\nabla} I \cdot \boldsymbol{w}) \boldsymbol{w}] \bar{I} d\boldsymbol{y}.\end{aligned} \tag{7}$$

Here, $\boldsymbol{\nu}$ is an outwardly directed normal vector at ∂Q which reduces to $\boldsymbol{n}$ at Γ. For the variational derivative above to vanish for all perturbations $\bar{I}$, in particular for perturbations vanishing on the boundary Γ, the following equation must hold in the interior:

$$\begin{aligned}\boldsymbol{\nabla} \cdot [(\boldsymbol{\nabla} I \cdot \boldsymbol{w}) \boldsymbol{w}] &= \nabla (\nabla I \cdot \boldsymbol{u} + I_z) \cdot \boldsymbol{u} + (\nabla I \cdot \boldsymbol{u} + I_z)_z + (\nabla \cdot \boldsymbol{u})(\nabla I \cdot \boldsymbol{u} + I_z) \\ &= \frac{d^2 I}{d\zeta^2} + (\nabla \cdot \boldsymbol{u}) \frac{dI}{d\zeta} = 0 \quad \text{in } Q\end{aligned} \tag{8}$$

in which (9) has been applied. Consider now the choice of boundary conditions shown in (2). For the boundary term in (7) to vanish for all perturbations $\bar{I}$, there are three possibilities on Γ: $\bar{I} = 0$, $\boldsymbol{u} \cdot \boldsymbol{n} = 0$, or $\boldsymbol{\nabla} I \cdot \boldsymbol{w} = 0$. The first case corresponds to having imposed (2) so that the perturbation $\bar{I}$ would be constrained to vanish on all of ∂Q. To see the unsatisfactory consequences of the other two options, consider first that $\boldsymbol{u} \cdot \boldsymbol{n} = 0$ is imposed at Γ. This means that trajectories would not be allowed to impinge upon the boundary at Γ, and this restriction would clearly corrupt a rigid registration. Since it is required to produce a rigid registration

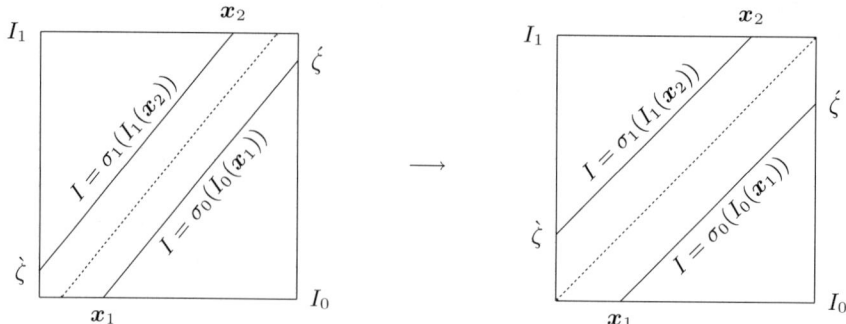

Fig. 2. When the intensity I is constant along trajectories connected with Γ, all trajectories are drawn toward Γ until the cost J vanishes.

when one fits the data, the boundary condition $\boldsymbol{u} \cdot \boldsymbol{n} = 0$ at Γ is ruled out. Now consider that $\nabla I \cdot \boldsymbol{w} = dI/d\zeta = 0$ is imposed at Γ. Then fix a trajectory which departs from Ω_0 and impinges on Γ at $\zeta = \acute{\zeta}$ as shown in Fig. 2.

From (8), the conditions on the trajectory that $d^2I/d\zeta^2 + (\nabla \cdot \boldsymbol{u})dI/d\zeta = 0$ for $0 < \zeta < \acute{\zeta}$, $I = \sigma_0(I_0)$ at $\zeta = 0$, and $dI/d\zeta = 0$ at $\zeta = \acute{\zeta}$ imply that I remains constant at $I = \sigma_0(I_0)$ along the trajectory. The situation is similar for trajectories that depart from Ω_1 and impinge upon Γ in the reverse direction. This is in fact a state toward which the solution $(I, \sigma_0, \sigma_1, \boldsymbol{u})$ would be drawn since it reduces the cost J. Specifically, when the intensity I is computed in this way, the optical flow $\boldsymbol{u}$ is drawn in its next iteration toward more trajectories that impinge upon Γ. Eventually all trajectories impinge upon Γ to give the minimum possible cost, and no like points in I_0 and I_1 are connected. Clearly, this is a solution to be avoided. Thus, the intensity field is assumed to satisfy the boundary conditions (2).

From (2) and (8), the optimal intensity I for fixed σ_0, σ_1, and $\boldsymbol{u}$ is given in a Lagrangian frame by:

$$I(\boldsymbol{x}(\boldsymbol{\xi},\zeta),\zeta) = \begin{cases} \sigma_0(I_0(\boldsymbol{\xi}))[1 - U(\boldsymbol{\xi},\zeta,1)] + \sigma_1(I_1(\boldsymbol{x}(\boldsymbol{\xi},1)))U(\boldsymbol{\xi},\zeta,1), & \boldsymbol{\xi} \in \Omega_0^c \\ \sigma_0(I_0(\boldsymbol{\xi}))[1 - U(\boldsymbol{\xi},\zeta,\acute{\zeta})], & \boldsymbol{x}(\boldsymbol{\xi},\acute{\zeta}) \in \Gamma, \boldsymbol{\xi} \in \Omega_0^i \\ \sigma_0(I_0(\boldsymbol{\xi})), & \boldsymbol{x}(\boldsymbol{\xi},\acute{\zeta}) \in \Xi, \boldsymbol{\xi} \in \Omega_0^i, \end{cases} \quad (9)$$

and:

$$I(\boldsymbol{y}(\boldsymbol{\eta},\zeta),\zeta) = \begin{cases} \sigma_1(I_1(\boldsymbol{\eta}))[1 - V(\boldsymbol{\eta},0,\zeta)] + \sigma_0(I_0(\boldsymbol{y}(\boldsymbol{\eta},0)))V(\boldsymbol{\eta},0,\zeta), & \boldsymbol{\eta} \in \Omega_1^c \\ \sigma_1(I_1(\boldsymbol{\eta}))[1 - V(\boldsymbol{\eta},\grave{\zeta},\zeta)], & \boldsymbol{y}(\boldsymbol{\eta},\grave{\zeta}) \in \Gamma, \boldsymbol{\eta} \in \Omega_1^i \\ \sigma_1(I_1(\boldsymbol{\eta})), & \boldsymbol{y}(\boldsymbol{\eta},\grave{\zeta}) \in \Xi, \boldsymbol{\eta} \in \Omega_1^i \end{cases} \quad (10)$$

in terms of quantities defined as follows. Here, Ω_0^c and Ω_0^i are the disjoint subsets of Ω_0 from which trajectories extend completely and incompletely, respectively, through the full depth of Q. Also, Ω_1^c and Ω_1^i are disjoint subsets of Ω_1 defined similarly. Let $\Xi \subset Q$ denote a set in which trajectories fail to be well defined, e.g., due to a singularity in the optical flow field. Define U and V by:

$$U(\boldsymbol{\xi},\zeta,\acute{\zeta}) = \begin{cases} \dfrac{\tilde{U}(\boldsymbol{\xi},\zeta) - \tilde{U}(\boldsymbol{\xi},0)}{\tilde{U}(\boldsymbol{\xi},\acute{\zeta}) - \tilde{U}(\boldsymbol{\xi},0)}, \\ 0, \quad \boldsymbol{x}(\boldsymbol{\xi},\acute{\zeta}) \in \Xi, \end{cases} \quad \tilde{U}(\boldsymbol{\xi},\zeta) = \int_{\zeta_0}^{\zeta} \exp\left[-\int_{\zeta_0}^{\varrho} \nabla \cdot \boldsymbol{u}(\boldsymbol{x}(\boldsymbol{\xi},\rho),\rho)d\rho\right] d\varrho, \tag{11}$$

for $\boldsymbol{\xi} \in \Omega_0$, $\zeta \in [0, \acute{\zeta}]$, and arbitrary $\zeta_0 \in [0, \acute{\zeta}]$, and:

$$V(\boldsymbol{\eta},\grave{\zeta},\zeta) = \begin{cases} \dfrac{\tilde{V}(\boldsymbol{\eta},1) - \tilde{V}(\boldsymbol{\eta},\zeta)}{\tilde{V}(\boldsymbol{\eta},1) - \tilde{V}(\boldsymbol{\eta},\grave{\zeta})}, \\ 0, \quad \boldsymbol{y}(\boldsymbol{\eta},\grave{\zeta}) \in \Xi, \end{cases} \quad \tilde{V}(\boldsymbol{\eta},\zeta) = \int_{\zeta_0}^{\zeta} \exp\left[-\int_{\zeta_0}^{\varrho} \nabla \cdot \boldsymbol{u}(\boldsymbol{y}(\boldsymbol{\eta},\rho),\rho)d\rho\right] d\varrho, \tag{12}$$

for $\boldsymbol{\eta} \in \Omega_1$, $\zeta \in [\grave{\zeta},1]$, and arbitrary $\zeta_0 \in [\grave{\zeta},1]$. Under a condition such as $\boldsymbol{u} \in W^{1,\infty}(Q) \subset C^{0,1}(\bar{Q})$ [35], trajectories are well defined by (4) and (5) and the singular set Ξ is empty [10]. On the other hand, it is not intended to rule out situations where the registration is correctly described by a discontinuous optical flow field which would occur for instance when an object is excised. Suppose that $\Xi \subset Q$ denotes the set where shocks develop in the optical flow field as seen below in Fig. 4. Then trajectories are defined up to the shock and the intensity is constant along such trajectories as shown in (9) and (10). At all other points in Q not accessible from trajectories (4) or (5) the intensity is zero.

4.2 Optimality Conditions for Scaling

Next, for fixed I and $\boldsymbol{u}$, consider the computation of σ_0 and σ_1. Now the term (10) appearing in (1) can be written in a Lagrangian frame as follows:

$$\int_Q [\nabla I \cdot \boldsymbol{u} + I_z]^2 d\boldsymbol{x}dz = T_0^c + T_0^i + T_1^i \equiv \int_{\Omega_0^c} \int_0^1 \left[\frac{dI}{d\zeta}\right]^2 \det(\nabla_{\boldsymbol{\xi}}\boldsymbol{x}) \, d\zeta d\boldsymbol{\xi} +$$

$$\int_{\Omega_0^i} \int_0^{\acute{\zeta}(\boldsymbol{\xi})} \left[\frac{dI}{d\zeta}\right]^2 \det(\nabla_{\boldsymbol{\xi}}\boldsymbol{x}) \, d\zeta d\boldsymbol{\xi} + \int_{\Omega_1^i} \int_{\grave{\zeta}(\boldsymbol{\eta})}^1 \left[\frac{dI}{d\zeta}\right]^2 \det(\nabla_{\boldsymbol{\eta}}\boldsymbol{y}) \, d\zeta d\boldsymbol{\eta} \tag{13}$$

where the first integral can be written equivalently with (10), (5), and (12) over Ω_1^c:

$$\int_{\Omega_0^c} \int_0^1 \left[\frac{dI}{d\zeta}\right]^2 \det(\nabla_{\boldsymbol{\xi}}\boldsymbol{x}) \, d\zeta d\boldsymbol{\xi} \equiv T_0^c = T_1^c \equiv \int_{\Omega_1^c} \int_0^1 \left[\frac{dI}{d\zeta}\right]^2 \det(\nabla_{\boldsymbol{\eta}}\boldsymbol{y}) \, d\zeta d\boldsymbol{\eta}. \tag{14}$$

Also, (9) and (10) define $\acute{\zeta}$ and $\grave{\zeta}$ as functions of $\boldsymbol{\xi}$ and $\boldsymbol{\eta}$, respectively, and can be used to express (13) and (14) explicitly in terms of σ_0 and σ_1:

$$T_0^c = \int_{\Omega_0^c} \int_0^1 [\sigma_0(I_0(\boldsymbol{\xi})) - \sigma_1(I_1(\boldsymbol{x}(\boldsymbol{\xi},1)))]^2 U_\zeta^2(\boldsymbol{\xi},\zeta,1) \det(\nabla_{\boldsymbol{\xi}}\boldsymbol{x}) \, d\zeta d\boldsymbol{\xi} \tag{15}$$

$$T_1^c = \int_{\Omega_0^c} \int_0^1 [\sigma_1(I_1(\eta)) - \sigma_0(I_0(y(\eta,0)))]^2 V_\zeta^2(\eta,0,\zeta) \det(\nabla_\eta y) \, d\zeta d\eta \quad (16)$$

$$T_0^i = \int_{\Omega_0^i} \int_0^{\acute{\zeta}(\xi)} \sigma_0^2(I_0(\xi)) U_\zeta^2(\xi,\zeta,\acute{\zeta}(\xi)) \det(\nabla_\xi x) \, d\zeta d\xi \quad (17)$$

$$T_1^i = \int_{\Omega_1^i} \int_{\grave{\zeta}(\eta)}^1 \sigma_1^2(I_1(\eta)) V_\zeta^2(\eta,\grave{\zeta}(\eta),\zeta) \det(\nabla_\eta y) \, d\zeta d\eta. \quad (18)$$

Since (17) and (18) are independent of σ_1 and σ_0, respectively, the variational derivative of J with respect to σ_0 for fixed σ_1 is:

$$\frac{\delta J}{\delta \sigma_0}(\sigma_0; \bar{\sigma}_0) = 2 \int_{\Omega_0} [\sigma_0(I_0(\xi)) - \mathcal{I}_1(\xi)] \bar{\sigma}_0(I_0(\xi)) \mathcal{U}(\xi) d\xi \quad (19)$$

and with respect to σ_1 for fixed σ_0 is:

$$\frac{\delta J}{\delta \sigma_1}(\sigma_1; \bar{\sigma}_1) = 2 \int_{\Omega_1} [\sigma_1(I_1(\eta)) - \mathcal{I}_0(\eta)] \bar{\sigma}_1(I_1(\eta)) \mathcal{V}(\eta) d\eta \quad (20)$$

where

$$\mathcal{U}(\xi) = \begin{cases} \int_0^1 U_\zeta^2(\xi,\zeta,1) \det(\nabla_\xi x) \, d\zeta, & \xi \in \Omega_0^c \\ \int_0^{\acute{\zeta}(\xi)} U_\zeta^2(\xi,\zeta,\acute{\zeta}(\xi)) \det(\nabla_\xi x) \, d\zeta, & \xi \in \Omega_0^i \end{cases} \quad (21)$$

$$\mathcal{V}(\eta) = \begin{cases} \int_0^1 V_\zeta^2(\eta,0,\zeta) \det(\nabla_\eta y) \, d\zeta, & \eta \in \Omega_1^c \\ \int_{\grave{\zeta}(\eta)}^1 V_\zeta^2(\eta,\grave{\zeta}(\eta),\zeta) \det(\nabla_\eta y) \, d\zeta, & \eta \in \Omega_1^i \end{cases} \quad (22)$$

and:

$$\mathcal{I}_0(\eta) = \begin{cases} \sigma_0(I_0(y(\eta,0))), & \eta \in \Omega_1^c \\ 0, & y(\eta,\grave{\zeta}) \in \Gamma, \eta \in \Omega_1^i \\ \sigma_1(I_1(\eta)), & y(\eta,\grave{\zeta}) \in \Xi, \eta \in \Omega_1^i \end{cases} \quad (23)$$

$$\mathcal{I}_1(\xi) = \begin{cases} \sigma_1(I_1(x(\xi,1))), & \xi \in \Omega_0^c \\ 0, & x(\xi,\acute{\zeta}) \in \Gamma, \xi \in \Omega_0^i \\ \sigma_0(I_0(\xi)), & x(\xi,\acute{\zeta}) \in \Xi, \xi \in \Omega_0^i. \end{cases} \quad (24)$$

Now let $\hat{\imath}_0 = \max\{I_0(\xi) : \xi \in \Omega_0\}$ and $\hat{\imath}_1 = \max\{I_1(\eta) : \eta \in \Omega_1\}$, so the ranges of I_0 and I_1 are $[0, \hat{\imath}_0]$ and $[0, \hat{\imath}_1]$. Then assume that $|\nabla I_0| = 0$ when I_0 assumes values $K_0 \subset [0, \hat{\imath}_0]$ and $|\nabla I_1| = 0$ when I_1 assumes values $K_1 \subset [0, \hat{\imath}_1]$. Further, let the integral in (19) be decomposed into the support of $|\nabla I_0|$ and its complement in Ω_0, and similarly let the integral in (20) be decomposed into the support of $|\nabla I_1|$ and its complement in Ω_1. Then, with the coarea formula [9], the variational derivatives take the forms:

$$\frac{\delta J}{\delta \sigma_0}(\sigma_0; \bar{\sigma}_0) = 2 \sum_{\iota \in K_0} \bar{\sigma}_0(\iota) \int_{I_0(\boldsymbol{\xi})=\iota} [\sigma_0(\iota) - \mathcal{I}_1(\boldsymbol{\xi})] \mathcal{U}(\boldsymbol{\xi}) d\boldsymbol{\xi}$$

$$+ 2 \int_0^{\hat{\iota}_0} \bar{\sigma}_0(\iota) \left[\int_{I_0(\boldsymbol{\xi})=\iota, \nabla I_0(\boldsymbol{\xi}) \neq 0} [\sigma_0(\iota) - \mathcal{I}_1(\boldsymbol{\xi})] \frac{\mathcal{U}(\boldsymbol{\xi})}{|\nabla I_0(\boldsymbol{\xi})|} d\boldsymbol{\xi} \right] d\iota \quad (25)$$

and:

$$\frac{\delta J}{\delta \sigma_1}(\sigma_1; \bar{\sigma}_1) = 2 \sum_{\iota \in K_1} \bar{\sigma}_1(\iota) \int_{I_1(\boldsymbol{\eta})=\iota} [\sigma_1(\iota) - \mathcal{I}_0(\boldsymbol{\eta})] \mathcal{V}(\boldsymbol{\eta}) d\boldsymbol{\eta}$$

$$+ 2 \int_0^{\hat{\iota}_1} \bar{\sigma}_1(\iota) \left[\int_{I_1(\boldsymbol{\eta})=\iota, \nabla I_1(\boldsymbol{\eta}) \neq 0} [\sigma_1(\iota) - \mathcal{I}_0(\boldsymbol{\eta})] \frac{\mathcal{V}(\boldsymbol{\eta})}{|\nabla I_1(\boldsymbol{\eta})|} d\boldsymbol{\eta} \right] d\iota. \quad (26)$$

Requiring these variational derivatives to vanish for all perturbations $\bar{\sigma}_0$ and $\bar{\sigma}_1$ leads to the following optimality conditions for σ_0 and σ_1:

$$\sigma_0(\iota) = \begin{cases} \int_{I_0(\boldsymbol{\xi})=\iota} \mathcal{I}_1(\boldsymbol{\xi}) \mathcal{U}(\boldsymbol{\xi}) d\boldsymbol{\xi} \Big/ \int_{I_0(\boldsymbol{\xi})=\iota} \mathcal{U}(\boldsymbol{\xi}) d\boldsymbol{\xi}, & \iota \in K_0, \\ \int_{I_0(\boldsymbol{\xi})=\iota} \mathcal{I}_1(\boldsymbol{\xi}) \frac{\mathcal{U}(\boldsymbol{\xi})}{|\nabla I_0(\boldsymbol{\xi})|} d\boldsymbol{\xi} \Big/ \int_{I_0(\boldsymbol{\xi})=\iota} \frac{\mathcal{U}(\boldsymbol{\xi})}{|\nabla I_0(\boldsymbol{\xi})|} d\boldsymbol{\xi}, & \iota \in [0, \hat{\iota}_0] \setminus K_0 \end{cases} \quad (27)$$

and:

$$\sigma_1(\iota) = \begin{cases} \int_{I_1(\boldsymbol{\eta})=\iota} \mathcal{I}_0(\boldsymbol{\eta}) \mathcal{V}(\boldsymbol{\eta}) d\boldsymbol{\eta} \Big/ \int_{I_1(\boldsymbol{\eta})=\iota} \mathcal{V}(\boldsymbol{\eta}) d\boldsymbol{\eta}, & \iota \in K_1, \\ \int_{I_1(\boldsymbol{\eta})=\iota} \mathcal{I}_0(\boldsymbol{\eta}) \frac{\mathcal{V}(\boldsymbol{\eta})}{|\nabla I_1(\boldsymbol{\eta})|} d\boldsymbol{\eta} \Big/ \int_{I_1(\boldsymbol{\eta})=\iota} \frac{\mathcal{V}(\boldsymbol{\eta})}{|\nabla I_1(\boldsymbol{\eta})|} d\boldsymbol{\eta}, & \iota \in [0, \hat{\iota}_1] \setminus K_1. \end{cases} \quad (28)$$

Although (27) and (28) are not considered numerically in the present work, their meaning can be elucidated by simple examples. First, assume that the given optical flow corresponds to a rigid transformation, $\boldsymbol{u} = \hat{\boldsymbol{u}}$, as shown in (9). Then $\nabla \cdot \hat{\boldsymbol{u}} = 0$ holds and it follows with (11) and (12) that $U_\zeta = 1$ and $V_\zeta = 1$ hold. A direct calculation with (5) gives $\det(\nabla_{\boldsymbol{\xi}} \hat{\boldsymbol{x}}) = 1$. Solving (5) with (9) gives $\hat{\boldsymbol{y}}(\boldsymbol{\eta}, \zeta) = R(1 - \zeta)(\boldsymbol{\eta} - \boldsymbol{a}) + \boldsymbol{a}$ and therefore $\det(\nabla_{\boldsymbol{\eta}} \hat{\boldsymbol{y}}) = 1$. Hence, with (21) and (22) it follows that $\mathcal{U} = 1$ and $\mathcal{V} = 1$ hold. Now for simplicity, assume that I_0 and I_1 are both equal to one on their supports which are contained strictly within Ω_0^c and Ω_1^c, respectively. Assume also that σ_0 and σ_1 are initialized as the identity. Then

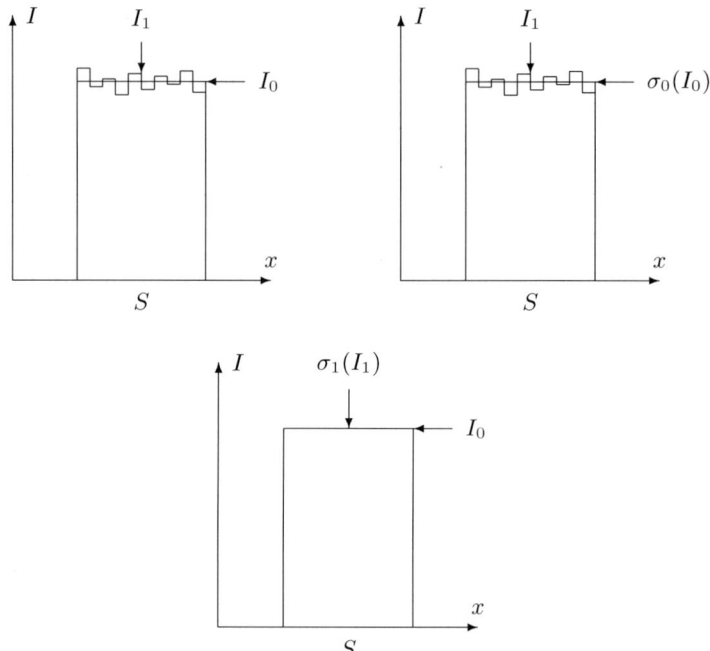

Fig. 3. Scaling I_0 without scaling I_1 leaves $\sigma_0(I_0)$ a binary image. Scaling I_1 without scaling I_0 gives $\sigma_1(I_1) = I_0$. Thus, the result of nonreciprocal scaling depends upon the order in which images are taken.

according to (27), the average of $I_1(x(\boldsymbol{\xi}, 1))$ over the support of $I_0(\boldsymbol{\xi})$ gives the value $\sigma_0(1)$. Similarly, with (27), the average of $I_0(y(\boldsymbol{\eta}, 0))$ over the support of $I_1(\boldsymbol{\eta})$ gives the value $\sigma_1(1)$. With a perfect registration, $\sigma_0(1) = \sigma_1(1) = 1$.

Now to illustrate the importance of scaling reciprocally, suppose that $u = 0$ for two images, shown in Fig. 3, which are identical except that I_1 is noisy and I_0 is not. For simplicity, assume for a square S, $I_0 = \chi_S$ and $I_1 = I_1 \chi_S$, where the characteristic function χ_S is equal to one on the support S. Assume now that no scaling is performed for I_1 so that $\sigma_1(\iota) = \iota$. Then, as explained above, $\sigma_0(1)$ is calculated as the average of I_1 over S. Specifically, $\sigma_0(I_0)$ remains a binary image while $\sigma_1(I_1) = I_1$ does not. Therefore, by (9), the intensity distribution $I(\boldsymbol{x}, z) = \sigma_0(I_0(\boldsymbol{x}))[1 - z] + I_1(\boldsymbol{x})z$ drives a disturbance in u in the next optical flow calculation. Assume now on the other hand, that no scaling is performed for I_0 so that $\sigma_0(\iota) = \iota$. Then since the average of I_0 on any subset of S is equal to one, the calculation of σ_1 gives $\sigma_1(I_1(\boldsymbol{x})) = I_0(\boldsymbol{x})$. Therefore, from (9) the intensity field $I(\boldsymbol{x}, z) = I_0(\boldsymbol{x})$ preserves the optical flow $u = 0$, unlike the case with scaling only on I_0. Thus, reciprocal scaling is required for the registration result to be independent of the order in which images are taken.

This example also shows the importance of initializing the scaling functions with the identity at each iteration, since otherwise the resolution of certain intensity values can be lost in all subsequent iterations.

4.3 Optimality Conditions for Optical Flow

Now, for fixed I, σ_0, and σ_1, the variational derivative of J with respect to u is given by:

$$\frac{\delta J}{\delta u}(u;\bar{u}) = 2\int_Q [(\nabla I \cdot u + I_z)(\nabla I \cdot \bar{u}) + \alpha(u_z \cdot \bar{u}_z)]\,dxdz$$

$$+ 2\int_Q \phi'\left(|\nabla u^T + \nabla u|^2\right)[\nabla u^T + \nabla u] : [\nabla \bar{u}^T + \nabla \bar{u}]\,dxdz. \quad (29)$$

The optical flow u is computed by solving the weakly formulated optimality system:

$$0 = \frac{1}{2}\frac{\delta J}{\delta u}(u;\bar{u}) = B(u,u,\bar{u}) - F(\bar{u}), \qquad \forall \bar{u} \in C^\infty(\bar{Q}), \quad (30)$$

where B and F are defined as follows:

$$B(u,v,w) = \int_Q [(\nabla I \cdot v)(\nabla I \cdot w) + \alpha(v_z \cdot w_z)]\,dxdz$$

$$+ \int_Q \phi'\left(|\nabla u^T + \nabla u|^2\right)(\nabla v^T + \nabla v) : (\nabla w^T + \nabla w)\,dxdz \quad (31)$$

$$F(w) = -\int_Q I_z \nabla I \cdot w\,dxdz. \quad (32)$$

The solvability of (30) is considered below in Theorem 2 for linear ϕ. The optimality system is also given below in differential form. As explained in connection with (7), only natural boundary conditions are considered for u in order to avoid disturbances to rigid registrations, and therefore, the above variational derivative satisfies

$$\frac{1}{2}\frac{\delta J}{\delta u}(u;\bar{u}) = \int_Q \Big\{(\nabla I \cdot u + I_z)\nabla I - \alpha u_{zz}$$
$$-\nabla \cdot \left[2\phi'\left(|\nabla u^T + \nabla u|^2\right)(\nabla u^T + \nabla u)\right]\Big\} \cdot \bar{u}\,dxdz$$
$$+ \int_\Gamma n \cdot \left[2\phi'\left(|\nabla u^T + \nabla u|^2\right)(\nabla u^T + \nabla u)\right] \cdot \bar{u}\,dxdz \quad (33)$$
$$+ \int_{\Omega_1} \alpha u_z \cdot \bar{u}\,dx - \int_{\Omega_0} \alpha u_z \cdot \bar{u}\,dx.$$

Requiring this variational derivative to vanish for smooth perturbations $\bar{u}$ which have vanishingly small support while remaining concentrated at a given point in a

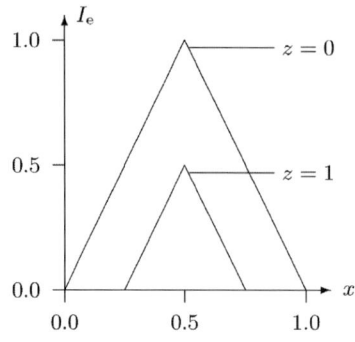 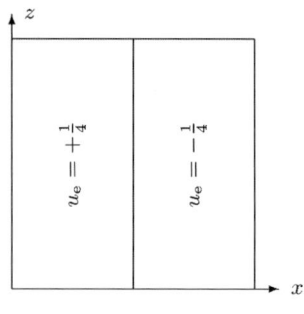

Fig. 4. The intensity I_e models the excision of an object from Ω_0, and the discontinuous u_e is the natural corresponding optical flow.

single integral above leads to the following optimality conditions on the optical flow u:

$$\begin{cases} -2\nabla \cdot \left[\phi' \left(|\nabla u^T + \nabla u|^2 \right) \left(\nabla u^T + \nabla u \right) \right] \\ \quad -\alpha u_{zz} + \left(\nabla I \nabla I^T \right) u = -I_z \nabla I, \quad Q, \\ n \cdot \left(\nabla u^T + \nabla u \right) = 0, \quad \Gamma, \qquad u_z = 0, \quad \Omega_0, \Omega_1. \end{cases} \quad (34)$$

To illustrate the effect of the function ϕ, consider the system for one-dimensional images, $I_e(x,0)$ and $I_e(x,1)$ from $I_e(x,z) = \max\{(1-\frac{1}{2}z) - 2|x-\frac{1}{2}|, 0\}$, which model the excision of an object $\{I_e(x,0) > \frac{1}{2}\}$ in Ω_0 as shown in Fig. 4. The natural corresponding optical flow is $u_e(x,z) = \frac{1}{4}\chi_{[0,1/2]}(x) - \frac{1}{4}\chi_{[1/2,1]}(x)$, but the corresponding cost is not finite if ϕ is linear. Instead, the fitting penalty in this case is total variation $\phi(s) = \beta\sqrt{s}$,

$$J(u) = \int_0^1 \int_{\frac{z}{4}}^{\frac{1}{2}} (2u - \tfrac{1}{2})^2 dx dz + \int_0^1 \int_{\frac{1}{2}}^{1-\frac{z}{4}} (2u + \tfrac{1}{2})^2 dx dz \\ + \int_0^1 \int_0^1 \left[2\beta |u_x| + \alpha |u_z|^2 \right] dx dz \quad (35)$$

for which $J(u_e) = \beta$ and for which (30) holds with $u = u_e$. Note the difficulty in implementing such singular transformations in a purely Lagrangian frame such as with (4). Of course, if smoother registrations are desired, then choosing a linear function ϕ is more appropriate. Intermediate regularization goals can be reached through intermediate choices for ϕ [39], but it is assumed here that $\phi(s^2)$ is convex for well-posed minimization [3].

4.4 Well-Posedness of the Variational Problem

It is not quite clear beforehand whether the cost function (1) is sufficiently coercive with respect to u to guarantee well-posedness for (30) or whether additional optical flow regularization such as

$$\int_Q \phi\left(|\nabla \boldsymbol{u}|^2\right) d\boldsymbol{x}dz \tag{36}$$

is necessary. For instance, suppose the intensity has the form $I(\boldsymbol{x}, z) = |\boldsymbol{x}|^2$ in Q, and thereby supports an ambiguous optical flow $\boldsymbol{u}_\theta = \theta W \boldsymbol{x}$ for any $\theta \in \boldsymbol{R}$ and for any skew-symmetric matrix $W \in \boldsymbol{R}^{N \times N}$. Then the cost is zero for every $\theta \in \boldsymbol{R}$, and in particular $J(\boldsymbol{u}_\theta) \not\to \infty$ as $\|\boldsymbol{u}_\theta\|_{H^1(Q)} = \mathcal{O}(\theta) \to \infty$. However, it can be assumed safely that medical images do not support such ambiguity. Thus, on the basis of the following theorem, the regularization shown in (36) is not used in this work.

Theorem 2. *Suppose that an intensity $I \in W^{1,\infty}(Q)$ manifests sufficiently few symmetries that for every $\boldsymbol{a} \in \boldsymbol{R}^N$ and for every skew-symmetric $W \in \boldsymbol{R}^{N \times N}$,*

$$\int_Q |\nabla I \cdot (\boldsymbol{a} + W\boldsymbol{x})|^2 d\boldsymbol{x}dz > 0, \tag{37}$$

unless $\boldsymbol{a} = 0 = W$. Then with $\phi(s) = \beta(\boldsymbol{x}, z)s$, $0 < \beta_0 \leq \beta(\boldsymbol{x}, z) \leq \beta_1 < \infty$, there exists a unique $\boldsymbol{u} \in H^1(Q)$ such that (30) holds.

Proof: Since $C^\infty(\bar{Q})$ is dense in $H^1(Q)$, the claim follows from the Lax-Milgram Theorem [6] once it is shown that $B(\boldsymbol{u}, \boldsymbol{v}) = B(\cdot, \boldsymbol{u}, \boldsymbol{v})$ is bounded and coercive on $H^1(Q)$ and that $F(\boldsymbol{v})$ is bounded on $H^1(Q)$. The boundedness of B and F is readily established:

$$|B(\boldsymbol{u}, \boldsymbol{v})| \leq \|I\|^2_{W^{1,\infty}(Q)} \|\boldsymbol{u}\|_{L^2(Q)} \|\boldsymbol{v}\|_{L^2(Q)} + \alpha \|\boldsymbol{u}_z\|_{L^2(Q)} \|\boldsymbol{v}_z\|_{L^2(Q)}$$
$$+ 4\beta_1 \|\nabla \boldsymbol{u}\|_{L^2(Q)} \|\nabla \boldsymbol{v}\|_{L^2(Q)}$$

$$\leq [\|I\|^2_{W^{1,\infty}(Q)} + \alpha + 4\beta_1] \|\boldsymbol{u}\|_{H^1(Q)} \|\boldsymbol{v}\|_{H^1(Q)} \tag{38}$$

$$|F(\boldsymbol{v})| \leq \|I\|^2_{W^{1,\infty}(Q)} \|\boldsymbol{v}\|_{L^2(Q)}. \tag{39}$$

To establish coercivity of B, assume there exists a sequence $\{\boldsymbol{u}_n\} \subset H^1(Q)$ such that

$$\|\boldsymbol{u}_n\|_{H^1(Q)} = 1 \quad \text{while} \quad B(\boldsymbol{u}_n, \boldsymbol{u}_n) \to 0. \tag{40}$$

For convenience, define now the semi-norm $|\cdot|_B$ satisfying the following inequality:

$$|\boldsymbol{u}|^2_B = \|\nabla \boldsymbol{u}^\mathrm{T} + \nabla \boldsymbol{u}\|^2_{L^2(Q)} + \|\boldsymbol{u}_z\|^2_{L^2(Q)} \leq \frac{1}{\min\{\alpha, \beta_0\}} B(\boldsymbol{u}, \boldsymbol{u}). \tag{41}$$

Since $H^1(Q)$ is compactly embedded in $L^2(Q)$ [1], there is a subsequence $\{\boldsymbol{u}_{n_l}\}$ which converges in $L^2(Q)$. From Korn's Inequality [32],

$$\|\nabla \boldsymbol{u}\|^2_{L^2(Q)} \leq k_1 \|\boldsymbol{u}\|^2_{L^2(Q)} + k_2 \|\nabla \boldsymbol{u}^\mathrm{T} + \nabla \boldsymbol{u}\|^2_{L^2(Q)} \tag{42}$$

5.2 Optical Flow Discretization

Now, consider the computation of the optical flow u from (34). The numerical approximation is obtained naturally from a finite element discretization of (29) [6]. Specifically, let $S_{h,\tau}$ be the space of tensor products of linear C^0 splines defined on Q, and let $u \in S_{h,\tau}$ be determined by:

$$B(u, u, \chi) = F(\chi), \qquad \forall \chi \in S_{h,\tau} \tag{5}$$

where B and F are given in (31) and (32). Because of the possible nonlinearity, ϕ' in (5), a lagged diffusivity iteration is used [38]. Specifically, given $u^{\ell-1} \in S_{h,\tau}$, let $u^\ell \in S_{h,\tau}$ be determined by:

$$B(u^{\ell-1}, u^\ell, \chi) = F(\chi), \qquad \forall \chi \in S_{h,\tau}. \tag{6}$$

For this, assume that ϕ is sufficiently regularized so that $0 < \beta_0 \leq \phi' \leq \beta_1 < \infty$. Thus, by Theorem 2, u^ℓ is well-defined by (6).

As illustrated in [19], finite element discretizations lead to aberrant consequences in the limit of vanishing regularization corresponding to an ever improving signal-to-noise ratio. To avoid these consequences as well as the wide bandwidth of the algebraic system in (6), a *lumping* approach is used to derive a finite difference discretization which is consistent with (6). Such lumping is implemented here by using cell-centered tensor products of spline basis functions:

$$s^{(0)}(t) = \chi_{[0,1]}(t), \quad s^{(1)}(t) = [s^{(0)} * s^{(0)}](t)$$

$$\begin{array}{ll} s^{(m_i)}(h^{-1}x_i - \mathbf{N} + \frac{m_i}{2}) \text{ on } Q_{x_i} = [\frac{m_i}{2}h, 1 - \frac{m_i}{2}h] \\ s^{(n)}(\tau^{-1}z - \mathbf{N} + \frac{n}{2}) \text{ on } Q_z = [\frac{n}{2}\tau, 1 - \frac{n}{2}\tau]. \end{array} \tag{7}$$

$$Q \approx \hat{Q} = Q_{x_1} \times \cdots \times Q_{x_N} \times Q_z$$

which are minimally smooth in a given direction for a given term as detailed below. The effect of this lumping is to concentrate the algebraic formulation at cell centers. Thus, the final system unknowns become the optical flow grid values directly instead of merely finite element basis function weights.

Lumping is implemented for the term $\int_{\hat{Q}} (\nabla I \cdot u)(\nabla I \cdot \chi) dx dz$ from $B(u^{\ell-1}, u, \chi)$ with $m_i = n = 0$ in (7) and leads to the algebraic coefficients $(\nabla I_{i,k} \nabla I_{i,k}^T) u_{i,k}$. Here, the numerical gradient $\nabla_h I$ is computed with simple central differences with natural one-sided modifications at the boundary. In spite of the apparent wavelike nature of the transport of intensities through Q, nonlinear gradient approximations [27] were not found necessary for the computation of $\nabla_h I$. The transport is however sensitive to the computation of I_z, which must be consistent with (9):

$$(I_z)_{i,k} = (dI/d\zeta)_{i,k} - \nabla_h I_{i,k} \cdot u_{i,k}^I \tag{8}$$

where u^I in (8) denotes the optical flow used to compute the intensity. With I_z computed in this way, the term $-\int_{\hat{Q}} I_z \nabla I \cdot \chi dx dz$ from $F(\chi)$ leads with $m_i = n = 0$ in (7) to the source term $-(I_z)_{i,k} \nabla_h I_{i,k}$.

Lumping is implemented as follows for the terms of $\int_{\hat{Q}} \phi'_{\ell-1}[(\nabla \boldsymbol{u}^\mathrm{T} + \nabla \boldsymbol{u}) :$
$(\nabla \boldsymbol{\chi}^\mathrm{T} + \nabla \boldsymbol{\chi})] d\boldsymbol{x} dz$ from $B(\boldsymbol{u}^{\ell-1}, \boldsymbol{u}, \boldsymbol{\chi})$. In all cases, $n = 0$ in (7). Then for diagonal terms, $\phi' \partial_{x_i} u_i \partial_{x_i} \chi_i$, the values $m_j = \delta_{ij}$ are used in (7). For off-diagonal terms, $\phi' \partial_{x_i} u_k \partial_{x_\iota} \chi_\kappa$, $i \neq \iota$, $k \neq \kappa$, the values $m_j = \delta_{ij} + \delta_{\iota j}$ are used in (7). Also,

$$\beta_{i,k} = \phi'\left(\left|[\nabla \boldsymbol{u}^\mathrm{T} + \nabla \boldsymbol{u}]_{i,k}^{\ell-1}\right|^2\right) \tag{9}$$

is computed using central differences for $\nabla \boldsymbol{u}^{\ell-1}$. Natural one-sided modifications are used at the boundary, and for fractional subscripts β is computed by differencing $\boldsymbol{u}^{\ell-1}$ symmetrically with respect to the appropriate cell face. This lumping is particularly useful to derive the numerical boundary conditions and the resulting stencils are given in detail in [20].

Finally, lumping is implemented for the term $\int_{\hat{Q}} \alpha[\boldsymbol{u}_z \cdot \boldsymbol{\chi}_z] d\boldsymbol{x} dz$ from $B(\boldsymbol{u}^{\ell-1}, \boldsymbol{u}, \boldsymbol{\chi})$ with $m_i = 0$ and $n = 1$ in (7), and leads to the standard finite difference discretization of the 1D Laplacian with Neumann boundary conditions.

The discretizations defined above lead to a $2^{N_p} K \times 2^{N_p} K$ linear system,

$$A_{\ell-1} \boldsymbol{u}^\ell = \boldsymbol{f} \tag{10}$$

in which the matrix $A_{\ell-1}$ is dependent upon $\boldsymbol{u}^{\ell-1}$. A detailed Taylor series analysis shows that this discretization is consistent with the differential form of the optimality system for the optical flow given in (34). According to the following, $\boldsymbol{u}^\ell$ is well defined by (10).

Theorem 4. *Suppose that the grid values $\{\nabla_h I_{i,k}\}$ manifest sufficiently few symmetries that for every $\boldsymbol{a} \in \boldsymbol{R}^N$ and for every skew-symmetric $W \in \boldsymbol{R}^{N \times N}$,*

$$\sum_{1 \leq i \leq 2^p \cdot 1} \sum_{1 \leq k \leq K} |\nabla_h I_{i,k} \cdot (\boldsymbol{a} + W \mathbf{x}_i)|^2 > 0, \tag{11}$$

unless $\boldsymbol{a} = 0 = W$. Also, assume that $\phi'_{\ell-1}$ is cellwise constant and that (9) satisfies $0 < \beta_0 \leq \beta_{i,k} \leq \beta_1 < \infty$. Then $A_{\ell-1}$ in (10) is a symmetric and positive definite matrix.

Proof: The matrix is evidently symmetric and non-negative. Suppose there exists a vector of grid values $\boldsymbol{u}^* = \{u^*_{i,k}\}$ such that $\boldsymbol{u}^* \cdot A_{\ell-1} \cdot \boldsymbol{u}^* = 0$.

Now let w represent the function which is cellwise constant with respect to x and piecewise linear and globally C^0 with respect to z, and suppose w has coefficients $\{u^*_{i,k}\}$ for the corresponding spline tensor products shown in (7). Then the terms in $\boldsymbol{u}^* \cdot A_{\ell-1} \cdot \boldsymbol{u}^*$ derived from integrals involving α result from substituting w in these integrals and thus,

$$0 = \boldsymbol{u}^* \cdot A_{\ell-1} \cdot \boldsymbol{u}^* \geq \int_{\hat{Q}} \alpha |w_z|^2. \tag{12}$$

Therefore, the coefficients $\{u^*_{i,k}\}$ are constant with respect to k.

Now let v represent the function which is cellwise constant with respect to z and piecewise multilinear and globally C^0 with respect to x, and suppose v has coefficients $\{u_{i,k}^*\}$ for the corresponding spline tensor products shown in (7). Then note that the mass matrices for $s^{(0)}(t)$ and $s^{(1)}(t)$, i.e.,

$$M^{(0)} = \left\{ \int_0^1 s^{(0)}(h^{-1}t - k)\, s^{(0)}(h^{-1}t - l)\, dt \, : \, 0 \leq k, l \leq h^{-1} \right\} \tag{13}$$

$$M^{(1)} = \left\{ \int_{\frac{h}{2}}^{1-\frac{h}{2}} s^{(1)}(h^{-1}t - k + \tfrac{1}{2}) s^{(1)}(h^{-1}t - l + \tfrac{1}{2}) dt : 0 \leq k, l \leq h^{-1} \right\} \tag{14}$$

satisfy the spectral property:

$$\tfrac{1}{6}\chi \cdot M^{(0)} \cdot \chi \leq \chi \cdot M^{(1)} \cdot \chi \leq \chi \cdot M^{(0)} \cdot \chi. \tag{15}$$

Therefore, all terms in $u^* \cdot A_{\ell-1} \cdot u^*$ derived from integrals involving $\phi'_{\ell-1}$ can be estimated in terms of tensor products of splines in (7) with $m_i = 1$ and $n = 0$. Thus, all such terms result from substituting v in the corresponding integrals and hence:

$$0 = u^* \cdot A_{\ell-1} \cdot u^* \geq \beta_0 \int_{\hat{Q}} |\nabla v^T + \nabla v|^2 dx dz. \tag{16}$$

Since the coefficients $\{u_{i,k}^*\}$ are constant with respect to k, v has the form $u_{i,k}^* = v(x_i, z_k) = a + W x_i$ for some $a \in R^N$ and for some skew-symmetric $W \in R^{N \times N}$, as argued in the proof of Theorem 2.

Finally, since $u^* \cdot A_{\ell-1} \cdot u^*$ majorizes the sum in (11), that sum must vanish. However, this violates the assumption on I unless $u^* = 0$. ∎

The computation of the optical flow can now be summarized as follows:
- Compute $\nabla_h I$ by central differences and I_z by (8).
- Set $u^0 = u$ and $\ell = 1$.
- Repeat until the relative difference in u^ℓ is sufficiently small:
  ○ Assemble $A_{\ell-1}$ using $u^{\ell-1}$, solve (10) for u^ℓ, and set $\ell = \ell + 1$.
- Set $u = u^\ell$.

According to Theorem 4, the system in (10) can be solved using a conjugate gradient method. Although conjugate gradient is relatively slow in the present context, it is used in the present work for convenience. On the other hand, note that if $\alpha = \infty$ ($u_z = 0$) and $\phi(s) = \beta s$, then (10) is ℓ-independent and has the spectral structure of the elasticity approach of [12] in which fast Fourier methods are used. However, particularly for the treatment of natural boundary conditions, the preferred solution procedure for (5) involves nonlinear multigrid techniques [16] [36] as well as multi-scale pyramidal strategies in place of the loop shown at the beginning of Section 5. Further numerical details will be reported separately.

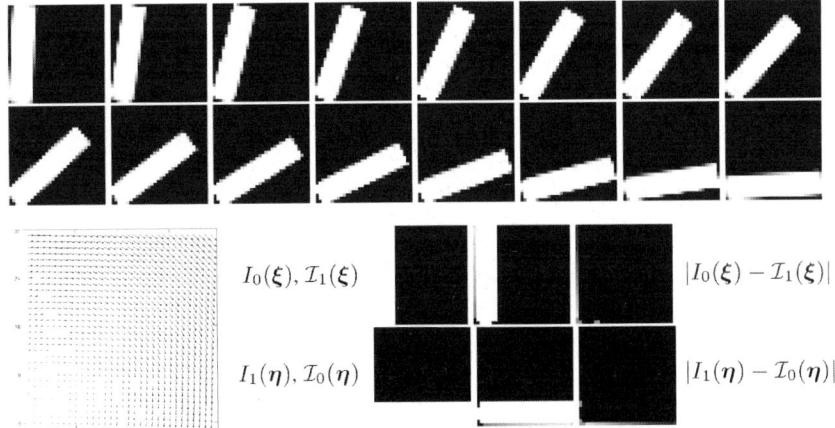

Fig. 8. In the two uppermost rows, the intermediate 32×32 images $\{\{I_{i,k}\} : 1 \leq k \leq 16\}$ are read from left to right and from top to bottom. The essentially z-independent computed optical flow field is shown in the lower left. The registration error is represented in the lower right, where $I_0(\xi), \mathcal{I}_1(\xi)$, and $|I_0(\xi) - \mathcal{I}_1(\xi)|$, respectively, appear in the top row, and $I_1(\eta)$, $\mathcal{I}_0(\eta)$, and $|I_1(\eta) - \mathcal{I}_0(\eta)|$, respectively, appear in the bottom row.

6 Computational Results

The final numerical methods defined in the previous section are applied first to test cases and then to magnetic resonance images. First, Fig. 8 shows a simple example in which the given 32×32 images I_0 and I_1, shown to the right of the optical flow vector field, are related by a pure rotation. All the computations reported in this section were performed using the IDL (See http://www.rsinc.com/idl/index.asp) (Interactive Data Language) system. In every example, h and τ are one but can be rescaled in terms of regularization parameters to be consistent with the definition $Q = (0,1)^N$. Also, $I \in [0,1]$ holds in all examples, and white represents $I = 1$ while black represents $I = 0$. In the example of Fig. 8, $\alpha = 10$ and $\phi(s) = \beta s$ with $\beta = 10$. The successful computation of the rotation is evident in the sequence of intermediate images $\{\{I_{i,k}\} : 1 \leq k \leq 16\}$ and in the essentially z-independent rotational optical flow field. Now with the transported or morphed images $\mathcal{I}_0$ and $\mathcal{I}_1$ defined in (23) and (24), define the registration errors:

$$E_0^p(\Omega) = \|I_0 - \mathcal{I}_1\|_{L^p(\Omega)}, \qquad \Omega \subseteq \Omega_0, \qquad (1)$$
$$E_1^p(\Omega) = \|\mathcal{I}_0 - I_1\|_{L^p(\Omega)}, \qquad \Omega \subseteq \Omega_1. \qquad (2)$$

For the example shown in Fig. 8, the errors satisfy $E_0^1(\Omega_0^c) = 0.0094 = E_1^1(\Omega_1^c)$ on the domain subsets on which trajectories extend completely through the full depth of Q, and $E_0^1(\Omega_0) = 0.014 = E_1^1(\Omega_1)$ on the full image domains. Also, $E_0^1(\Omega_0) = 0.016 = E_1^1(\Omega_1)$ holds for the example shown in Fig. 7 for which $\alpha = 1$ and $\beta = 1$ were used. Thus, the approach succeeds to produce a rotation or a translation when one fits the data.

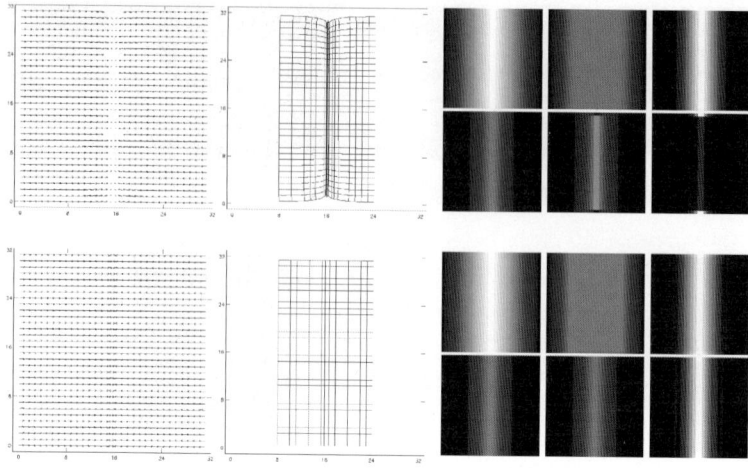

Fig. 9. Penalties $\phi(s) = \beta s$ and $\phi(s) = \beta\sqrt{s+\varepsilon}$ are compared in the top and bottom rows, respectively. The essentially k-independent optical flow fields are shown in the left column. The middle column shows the morphing of a uniform grid from Ω_0 to Ω_1. The corresponding registration errors are shown to the right in the same format as used in Fig. 8 but with scaled errors in the rightmost column. Specifically, for each penalty, $\mathcal{I}_0(\boldsymbol{\xi})$, $\mathcal{I}_1(\boldsymbol{\xi})$, and $|\mathcal{I}_0(\boldsymbol{\xi}) - \mathcal{I}_1(\boldsymbol{\xi})|/E_0^\infty(\Omega_0)$ appear above $\mathcal{I}_1(\boldsymbol{\eta})$, $\mathcal{I}_0(\boldsymbol{\eta})$, and $|\mathcal{I}_1(\boldsymbol{\eta}) - \mathcal{I}_0(\boldsymbol{\eta})|/E_1^\infty(\Omega_1)$, respectively.

On the other hand, the example shown in Fig. 8 is also constructed so that trajectories emanating from nontrivial pixels in Ω_0 and Ω_1 would impinge on the boundary Γ. As a result, the registration error satisfies $E_0^\infty(\Omega_0^c) = 0.52 = E_1^\infty(\Omega_1^c)$ on the subdomains Ω_0^c and Ω_1^c, but $E_0^\infty(\Omega_0) = 1 = E_1^\infty(\Omega_1)$ on the full domains Ω_0 and Ω_1. By contrast $E_0^\infty(\Omega_0) = 0.45 = E_1^\infty(\Omega_1)$ holds for the translation example shown in Fig. 7. Although the desired registration has been computed for the rotation, there is clearly a potentially influential loss of information when nontrivial trajectories impinge upon Γ, and such a loss can be avoided simply by extending images by zero and using a sufficiently large domain. The alternative use of non-natural boundary conditions would clearly disturb the images shown in Fig. 8.

Next, Fig. 9 shows a computational counterpart to Fig. 4 in which the given 32×32 images I_0 and I_1 are related by an excision, i.e., the middle component $\{I_0 > \frac{1}{2}\}$ is removed to create I_1. According to the same format used in Fig. 8, I_0 appears above I_1 leftmost among the images shown in Fig. 9. Also, the (Gaussian) penalty $\phi(s) = \beta s$, $\beta = 10^{-3}$, and the (regularized TV) penalty $\phi(s) = \beta\sqrt{s+\varepsilon}$, $\beta = 10^{-4}, \varepsilon = 10^{-2}$ are compared. In both cases, $K = 4$ and $\alpha = 10^5$ are chosen, and the optical flow field is essentially k-independent. The superior performance of the TV penalty can be seen most conspicuously from the middle column in Fig. 9 which shows a morphing of a uniform grid from Ω_0 to Ω_1. Note that for both penalties, the wide grey zone in $\mathcal{I}_1$ shows that the middlemost region of I_1 has been expanded. On the other hand, while the TV penalty maps only greyer pixels in I_0

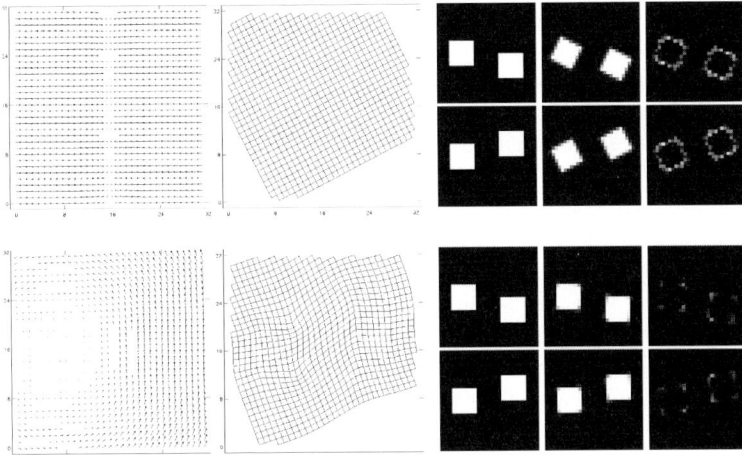

Fig. 10. To demonstrate strongly and weakly rigid registration with a simple example, penalties $\phi(s) = \beta s$ with large and small β are compared in the top and bottom rows, respectively. The essentially k-independent optical flow fields are shown in the left column. The middle column shows the morphing of a uniform grid from Ω_0 to Ω_1. The corresponding registration errors are shown to the right in the same format as used in Fig. 8 but with scaled errors in the rightmost column. Specifically, for each penalty, $\mathcal{I}_0(\boldsymbol{\xi}), \mathcal{I}_1(\boldsymbol{\xi})$, and $|\mathcal{I}_0(\boldsymbol{\xi}) - \mathcal{I}_1(\boldsymbol{\xi})|/E_0^\infty(\Omega_0)$ appear above $\mathcal{I}_1(\boldsymbol{\eta}), \mathcal{I}_0(\boldsymbol{\eta})$, and $|\mathcal{I}_1(\boldsymbol{\eta}) - \mathcal{I}_0(\boldsymbol{\eta})|/E_1^\infty(\Omega_1)$, respectively.

onto $\mathcal{I}_0$, the Gaussian penalty spuriously maps some brighter pixels of $\mathcal{I}_0$ onto $\mathcal{I}_0$ to generate a brighter strip in the middle of $\mathcal{I}_0$. Also, the inappropriate x_2-dependence resulting from the Gaussian penalty, particularly in the top and bottom image borders, is evident in the corresponding images $\mathcal{I}_0$ and $|I_1 - \mathcal{I}_0|/E_1^\infty(\Omega_1)$. With the Gaussian penalty, the errors are $E_0^1(\Omega_0^c) = 0.14$, $E_0^\infty(\Omega_0^c) = 0.5$, $E_1^1(\Omega_1^c) = 0.011$, and $E_1^\infty(\Omega_1^c) = 0.29$ on the subdomains, and $E_0^1(\Omega_0) = 0.14$, $E_0^\infty(\Omega_0) = 0.5$, $E_1^1(\Omega_1) = 0.013$, and $E_1^\infty(\Omega_1) = 0.5$ on the full domains. With the TV penalty, the errors are $E_0^1 = 0.14$, $E_0^\infty = 0.5$, $E_1^1 = 0.005$, and $E_1^\infty = 0.025$ both on the subdomains and the full domains.

Now, Fig. 10 shows a final simple example to reveal how the strongly rigid registration shown especially in Fig. 8 can be relaxed to what will be referred to as weakly rigid registration obtained by relaxing the dominance of the rigidity penalty. Again, following the format of Figs. 8 and 9, I_0 is shown above I_1 leftmost among the images shown in Fig. 10. Here, the 32×32 images I_0 and I_1 both contain a left-situated square which remains fixed, while a right-situated square moves upward from I_0 to I_1. In both cases of this example, a linear penalty, $\phi(s) = \beta s$, is used and $K = 2$ and $\alpha = 10$ are chosen. The compared cases correspond to $\beta = 10$ (strongly rigid) in the upper part of Fig. 10 and to $\beta = 10^{-2}$ (weakly rigid) in the lower part. The difference between strongly and weakly rigid registration is particularly evident in the respective uniform grid morphings from Ω_0 to Ω_1 shown in the middle column of Fig. 10. Specifically, weakly rigid registration evidently permits a departure from rigidity, i.e., a fluctuation in areas and angles, which vanishes on average and with increasing variance as the dominance of the rigidity penalty is relaxed. The errors corresponding to the strongly rigid case are $E_0^1 = 0.037 = E_1^1$ and $E_0^\infty = 1 = E_1^\infty$ both on the subdomains and the full domains. The errors corresponding to the weakly rigid case are $E_0^1 = 0.0045 = E_1^1$ and $E_0^\infty = 0.41 = E_1^\infty$ both on the subdomains and the full domains. Note that this and other more complex examples were constructed particularly to generate a nonautonomous optical flow field. The field can of course be made nonautonomous for sufficiently small α, but the result manifests more numerical fluctuation than any information rich variation which contributes to the registration. The trend of the flows is toward autonomy, and suggests further investigation of the regularization discussed in Section 3.

Finally, Fig. 11 shows an example of the registration of two magnetic resonance images I_0 and I_1 from a contrast enhanced dynamic scan containing 128×128 pixels each. The scan was performed with a T1-weighted inversion recovery turbo-flash sequence. Again, following the format of Figs. 8 – 10, I_0 is shown above I_1 leftmost among the images shown in Fig. 11. The most conspicuous object in the middle of these images is the left kidney situated to the right of the vertebral column appearing along the left border. This example is similar to that of Fig. 10 in the sense that the left-situated vertebrae remain fixed while the right-situated kidney moves upward from I_0 to I_1 as a consequence of respiration. In both cases of this example, a linear penalty, $\phi(s) = \beta s$, is used and $K = 2$ and $\alpha = 10$ are chosen. As with Fig. 10, the compared cases correspond to $\beta = 10$ (strongly rigid) in the left part of Fig. 11 and to $\beta = 10^{-2}$ (weakly rigid) in the right part. The difference between strongly and weakly rigid registration is again particularly evident in the respective uniform grid morphings from Ω_0 to Ω_1 shown in the middle row of Fig. 11. The errors corresponding to the strongly rigid case are $E_0^1(\Omega_0^c) = 0.046$, $E_0^\infty(\Omega_0^c) = 0.58$, $E_1^1(\Omega_1^c) = 0.046$, and $E_1^\infty(\Omega_1^c) = 0.55$ on the subdomains, and $E_0^1(\Omega_0) = 0.049$, $E_0^\infty(\Omega_0) = 0.61$, $E_1^1(\Omega_1) = 0.048$, and $E_1^\infty(\Omega_1) = 0.62$ on the full domains. The errors corresponding to the weakly rigid case are $E_0^1(\Omega_0^c) = 0.030$, $E_0^\infty(\Omega_0^c) = 0.40$, $E_1^1(\Omega_1^c) = 0.029$, and $E_1^\infty(\Omega_1^c) = 0.44$ on the subdomains, and $E_0^1(\Omega_0) = 0.031$, $E_0^\infty(\Omega_0) = 0.43$, $E_1^1(\Omega_1) = 0.029$, and $E_1^\infty(\Omega_1) = 0.47$ on the full domains. The error images have been displayed according to a common scale, in which 0.64 represents the brightest error intensity, in order to reveal the improvement obtained by the weakly in relation to the strongly rigid registration. Note that these images were taken in sequence after the injection of a Gadolinium-DTPA based contrast agent, as is particularly evident from certain bright spots which appear suddenly in one image and not the other. The registration is particularly difficult in the neighborhood of a bright spot in I_1 situated to the left among the vertebrae, and forthcoming work on image similarity measures will be useful for treating such situations. The applications of primary interest for forthcoming research will be focused mainly on the registration of dynamic magnetic resonance imaging data, particularly for the study of tissues or organs with physiological motion such as the kidneys or the heart.

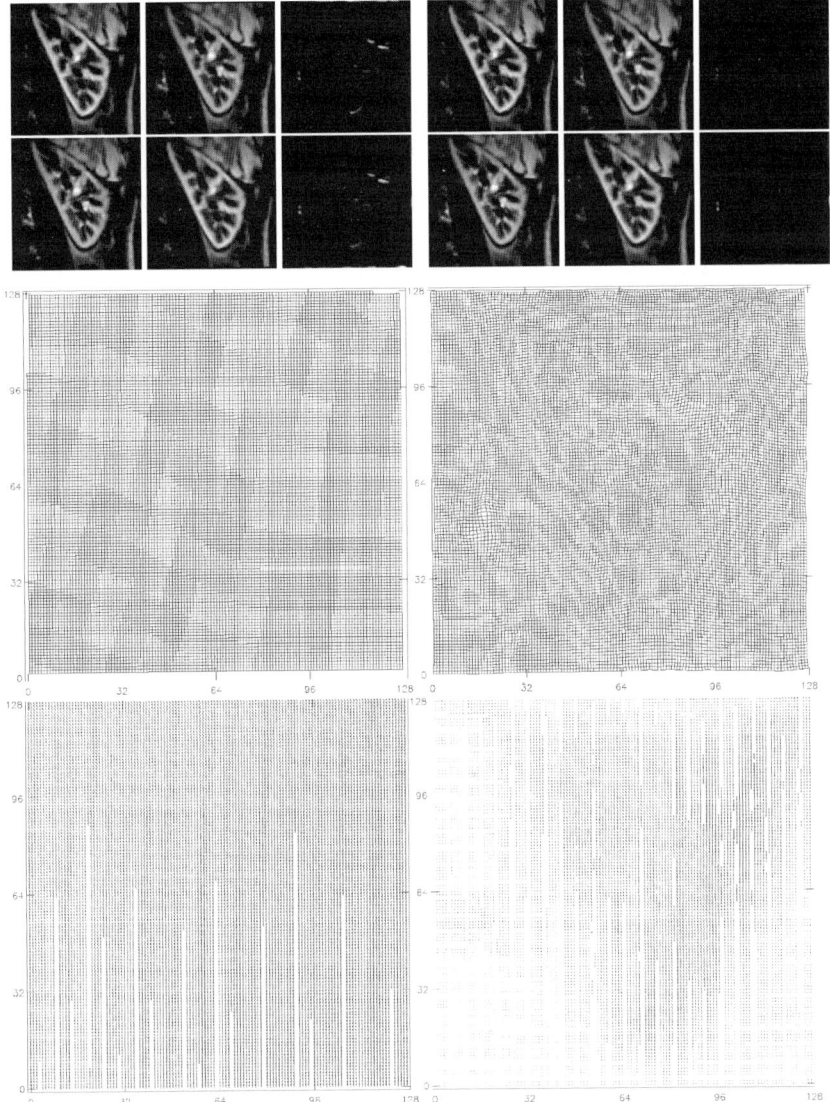

Fig. 11. To demonstrate strongly and weakly rigid registration of magnetic resonance images, penalties $\phi(s) = \beta s$ with large and small β are compared in the left and right columns, respectively. The essentially k-independent optical flow fields are shown in the bottom row. The middle row shows the morphing of a uniform grid from Ω_0 to Ω_1. The corresponding registration errors are shown at the top in the same format as used in Fig. 8 but with a common scale for the errors. Specifically, for each penalty, $I_0(\boldsymbol{\xi})$, $\mathcal{I}_1(\boldsymbol{\xi})$, and $|I_0(\boldsymbol{\xi}) - \mathcal{I}_1(\boldsymbol{\xi})|/0.64$ appear above $I_1(\boldsymbol{\eta})$, $\mathcal{I}_0(\boldsymbol{\eta})$, and $|I_1(\boldsymbol{\eta}) - \mathcal{I}_0(\boldsymbol{\eta})|/0.64$, respectively.

References

1. R.A. Adams: Sobolev Spaces, Academic Press, New York, (1975)
2. A. Borzi, K. Ito and K. Kunisch: Optimal Control Formulation for Determining Optical Flow, SIAM J. Sci. Comp., **24/3**, pp 818-847, (2002)
3. P. Charbonnier, F. Blanc-Féraud, G. Aubert and M. Barlaud: Deterministic Edge-Preserving Regularization in Computed Imaging, IEEE Trans. on Image Processing, **6/2** (1997)
4. D.R.J. Chillingworth: Differential Topology with a View to Applications, Pitman, London, (1976)
5. G. E. Christensen and H. J. Johnson: Consistent Image Registration, IEEE Trans. Med. Imaging. **20/7**, pp 568-582, (2001)
6. P.G. Ciarlet: The Finite Element Method for Elliptic Problems, North-Holland, Amsterdam, (1978)
7. P.G. Ciarlet: Mathematical Elasticity. Volume I: Three-Dimensional Elasticity, **20**, Studies in Mathematics and its Applications, North-Holland, Amsterdam, (1988)
8. P.G. Ciarlet: Mathematical Elasticity. Volume II: Theory of Plates, **27**, Studies in Mathematics and its Applications, North-Holland, Amsterdam, (1997)
9. L. C. Evans and R. F. Gariepy: Measure Theory and Fine Properties of Functions, CRC Press, Boca Raton, (1992)
10. H.O. Fattorini: Infinite Dimensional Optimization and Control Theory, Cambridge University Press, Cambridge, (1999)
11. B. Fischer and J. Modersitzki: Curvature Based Image Registration, J. Math. Imaging and Vision, **18**, pp 81-85, (2003)
12. B. Fischer and J. Modersitzki: Fast Inversion of Matrices Arising in Image Processing, Numerical Algorithms, **22**, pp 1-11, (1999)
13. M. Fitzpatrick, D. L. G. Hill and C. R. Maurer Jr.: Image Registration, Medical Image Processing, Chapter 8 of Volume II of the Handbook of Medical Imaging, M. Sonka and J.M. Fitzpatrick, ed., SPIE Press (July 2000).
14. M. Fitzpatrick, J. B. West, and C. R. Maurer Jr.: Predicting Error in Rigid-Body Point-Based Registration, IEEE Trans. Med. Imaging, **17**, pp 694-702, (1998)
15. S. Haker, A. Tannenbaum and R. Kikinis: Mass Preserving Mappings and Image Registration, MICCAI, pp 120-127, (2001)
16. S. Henn: Schnelle elastische Anpassung in der digitalen Bildverarbeitung mit Hilfe von Mehrgitterverfahren, Diplomarbeit Heinrich-Heine-Universität Düsseldorf, (1997)
17. W. Hinterberger: Generierung eines Films zwischen zwei Bildern mit Hilfe des optischen Flusses, Diplomarbeit, Institut für Industriemathematik der Technisch- Naturwissenschaftlichen Fakultät der Johannes Kepler Universität Linz, Linz, (Sept 1999)
18. B.K.P. Horn and B.G.Schunck: Determining Optical Flow, Artif. Intell., **23**, pp 185-203, (1981)
19. S.L. Keeling, R. Bammer: A Variational Approach to Magnetic Resonance Coil Sensitivity Estimation, Applied Mathematics and Computation, Vol. 158, No. 2, pp 53-82, (2004)
20. S. L. Keeling and W. Ring: Medical Image Registration and Interpolation by Optical Flow with Maximal Rigidity, SFB Report No. 248, Karl-Franzens-University of Graz, Graz, Austria, (May 2003)
21. M. Lefébure and L. D. Cohen: Image Registration, Optical Flow and Local Rigidity, J. Math. Imaging and Vision, **14/2**, pp 131-147, (March 2001)

22. J.A. Little, D.L.G. Hill and D.J. Hawkes: Deformations Incorporating Rigid Structures, Computer Vision and Image Understanding, **66/2**, pp 223-232, (1997)
23. D. G. Luenberger: Optimization by Vector Space Methods, John Wiley & Sons, Inc., New York, (1969)
24. F. Maes, A. Collignon, D. Vandermeulen, G. Marchal and P. Suetens: Multimodality Image Registration by Maximization of Mutual Information, IEEE Trans. Med. Imaging, **16**, pp 187-109, (1997)
25. J. Modersitzki: Numerical Methods for Image Registration, Oxford University Press, Oxford, (2004)
26. P. J. Olver: Applications of Lie Groups to Differential Equations, Springer, New York, (1986)
27. S. Osher and L. I. Rudin: Feature-Oriented Image Enhancement Using Shock Filters, SIAM J. Numer. Anal., **27/4**, pp 919-940, (August 1990)
28. W. Peckar, C. Schnörr, K. Rohr and H. S. Stiehl: Parameter-Free Elastic Deformation Approach for 2D and 3D Registration using Prescribed Displacements, J. Math. Imaging and Vision, **10**, pp 143-162, (1999)
29. D. Rueckert, B. Clarkson, D. L. G. Hill and D. J. Hawkes: Non-rigid Registration using Higher-Order Mutual Information, Medical Imaging 2000: Image Processing, K. M. Hanson, ed., Proceedings of SPIE, **3979**, pp 438-447, (2000)
30. D. Rueckert, L. I. Sonoda, C. Hayes, D.L.G. Hill, M. O. Leach and D.J. Hawkes: Non-rigid Registration using Free-Form Deformations: Application to Breast MR Images, IEEE Trans. Med. Imaging, **18/8**, pp 712-721, (1999)
31. C. Studholme, D. L. G. Hill and D. J. Hawkes: An Overlap Invariant Entropy Measure of 3D Medical Image Alignment, Pattern Recognition, **32**, pp 71-86, (1999)
32. M.E. Taylor: Partial Differential Equations: Basic Theory, Springer, New York, (1996)
33. J.-P. Thirion: Image Matching as a Diffusion Process: An Analogy with Maxwell's Demons, Medical Image Analysis, **2/3**, pp 243-260, (1998)
34. P.M. Thompson, M. S. Mega, K. L. Narr, E. R. Sowell, R. E. Blanton and A. W. Toga: Brain Image Analysis and Atlas Construction, Medical Image Processing, Chapter 17 of Volume II of the Handbook of Medical Imaging, M. Sonka and J.M. Fitzpatrick, ed., SPIE Press (July, 2000).
35. G.M. Troianiello: Elliptic differential equations and obstacle problems, Plenum Press, New York, (1987)
36. U. Trottenberg, C. Oosterlee and A. Schüller: Multigrid, Academic Press, San Diego, (2001)
37. P. A. Viola: Alignment by Maximization of Mutual Information., Ph.D. thesis, Massachusetts Institute of Technology, (1995)
38. C. R. Vogel and M. E. Oman: Iterative Methods for Total Variation Denoising, SIAM Journal on Scientific Computing, **17**, pp 227-238, (1996)
39. J. Weickert: Anisotropic Diffusion in Image Processing, B. G. Teubner Stuttgart, (1998)
40. W. M. Wells, P. Viola, H. Atsumi, S. Nakajima and R. Kikinis: Multi-modal Volume Registration by Maximization of Mutual Information, Med. Image Anal., **1**, 35-51, (1996)
41. J. B. West, J. M. Fitzpatrick, M. J. Wang, B.M. Dawant, C. R. Maurer Jr., R. M. Kessler, R. J. Maciunas, C. Barillot, D. Lemoine, A. Collignon, F. Maes, P. Suetens, D. Vandermeulen, P. A. van den Elsen, S. Napel, T. S. Sumanaweera, B. Harkness, P. F. Hemler, D. L. G. Hill, D. J. Hawkes, C. Studholme, J. B. A. Maintz, M. A. Viergever, G. Malandain, X. Pennec, M. E. Noz, G. Q. Maguire Jr., M. Pollack, C. A. Pelizzari, R. A. Robb, D. Hanson, R. P. Woods: Comparison and Evaluation of Retrospective Intermodality Brain Image Registration Techniques, J. Comput. Assist. Tomogr., **21**, pp 554-566, (1997)

Registration of Histological Serial Sectionings

Jan Modersitzki[1], Oliver Schmitt[2], and Stefan Wirtz[1]

[1] University of Lübeck, Institute of Mathematics, Wallstraße 40 D-23560 Lübeck
{modersitzki,wirtz}@math.uni-luebeck.de
[2] University of Rostock, Institute of Anatomy, Gertrudenstraße 9, D-18055 Rostock, Germany schmitt@med.uni-rostock.de

Summary Image registration is a fundamental task in today's medical imaging. In particular for histological serial sectioning, where a three-dimensional object is cut into thin sections for a further microscopic analysis, registration leads to a three dimensional reconstruction of the sections. This reconstruction enables an exploration of the digitized data in any direction, not only in the cutting direction. In this paper, we describe cutting and reconstruction procedures. For the reconstruction, we use linear as well as non-linear registration schemes. Moreover, we present some results for a whole brain of a *Sprague Dawley* rat.

1 Introduction

Histological serial sectioning is a valuable and essential tool in visualizing microscopic structures of tissue like, for example, cells. A three-dimensional object is sectioned into thin (5–40 μm) sections; cf. Fig. 1. These sections form the basis for a microscopic investigation; cf. Fig. 2. It is important to note that the sections are inevitable to deduce information about cells like, for example, size, position, and orientation. Alternative three-dimensional imaging devices like, for example, computer tomography (CT) or (micro) magnetic resonance imaging (MRI or μMRI) have resolutions that are far behind the visualization of cells [4, 11]. The information obtained from the microscopic analysis is related to the coordinates in the two-dimensional tissue section rather than the ones of the three-dimensional original object. However, the sectioning process introduces all kinds of deformations to the tissue and this results in distorted tissue sections; cf. Fig. 1(b). Therefore, the two-dimensional information can not be used to perform an overall three-dimensional analysis and visualization.

A remedy is provided by so-called image registration techniques; cf., e.g., [24, 17]. Image registration is one of the fundamental tasks in today's image processing and is used routinely in many medical applications; for an overview, see, e.g., [6, 16, 22, 17] and references therein. The objective of image registration is to make images which are taken at different times, from different perspectives, and/or from different devices to be more alike.

Particularly in the context of histological serial sectioning, the aim is to recover non-deformed versions of the tissue sections. Ideally, these non-deformed sections can then be glued together to get a three-dimensional tissue back; see also [19, 8, 21, 2]. By knowing the deformations, one can map from the deformed to the non-deformed tissue and vice versa. Therefore, one can also visualize cells in a three-dimensional view and perform a three-dimensional structure analysis.

Here, we describe a registration procedure for images arising in the Human NeuroScanning Project (HNSP) [23]. The overall goal of this project is a three-dimensional reconstruction of a whole human brain down to particular neurons based on microscopic modalities. This data will then be used as the basic structure for the integration of functional data based on stochastic mapping and later on for modelling and simulation studies in a virtual brain; see [23] for details.

The production of the histological serial sectioning of a human brain is addressed in Section 2. As illustrated in Fig. 3, non-linear registration is essential for the reconstruction of the brain sections. Fig. 3(a,b) displays two flat bed scans of consecutive sections of a serial sectioning of a human brain. The scans have been pre-registered using a principal axis transformation; cf., e.g., [1]. As it is apparent from the difference image Fig. 3(c), intolerable differences with respect to the geometry are observable (particularly near the cerebral cortex). Fig. 3(d) shows the difference after an affine linear registration. Though the difference has been reduced considerably and especially with respect to the left hemisphere, the result is still not convincing since large deformations are observable (particularly in the right hemisphere). This example demonstrates that the deformations to be observed are in general non-linear and therefore non-linear registration techniques have to be used in addition. Fig. 3(e) finally displays the difference image after an additional so-called elastic registration of these two slices. For elastic registration, we refer to the extended literature; see, e.g., [5, 3, 7, 10, 9, 12, 17].

The remaining part of the paper is organized as follows. In Section 3 we describe the three phases of our registration scheme. The first phase is related to some preprocessing: digitizing the tissue sections, segmentation, principal axis transformation (PAT) based pre-registration of the images (cf., e.g., [1]), and gray value equalization. The second phase is an affine linear registration of the image stack and the last phase is an elastic registration thereof.

Section 4 presents some results, the reconstruction and visualization of a whole brain of a *Sprague Dawley* rat. Moreover, we also present some timings for these particular reconstructions. Finally, we conclude in Section 5 and comment on future work.

2 Material

In order to locate the spatial positions of single neurons, the postmortem brain from a 55 year old male human voluntary donor was prepared in several steps; cf. [23]. In the beginning, the brain was fixed in a neutral buffered formaldehyde solution. After fixation an MR-scan of the brain was produced to obtain information of the original topology; cf. Fig. 2(a). Finally, the brain was dehydrated and embedded in paraffin; cf. Fig. 1(a).

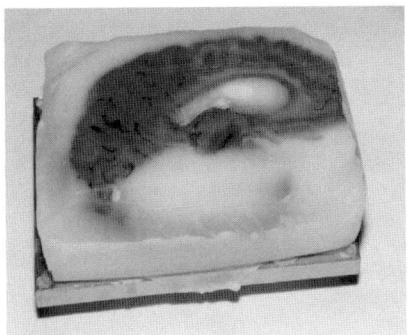
(a) paraffine embedded human brain (sagittal sectioning)

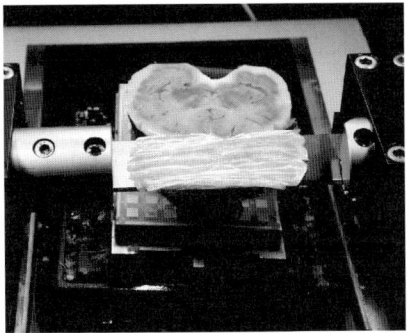
(b) sliding microtome with tissue section on the blade (axial sectioning)

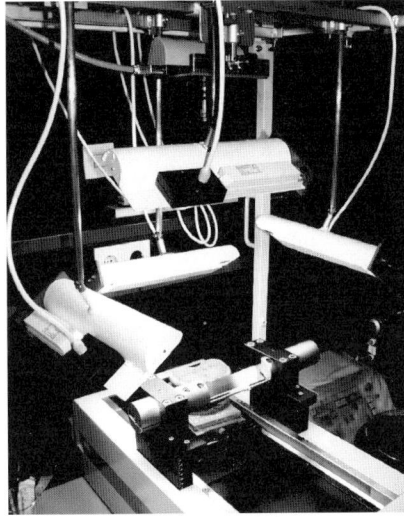
(c) slicing workbench

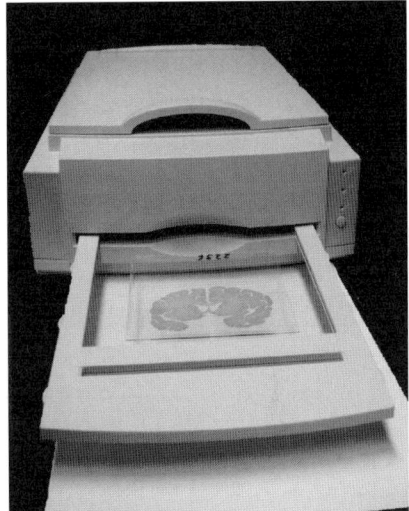
(d) high resolution FBS

Fig. 1. Sectioning machinery: (a) paraffin embed human brain; (b) sliding microtome with tissue section on top of the blade; (c) part of the slicing workbench; (d) transparent flat-bed-scanner (FBS) with microscopic slide.

This preparatory work was followed by sectioning the brain in 20 μm thick slices (about 5000 for this brain) using a sliding microtome; cf. Fig. 1(b,c). A high resolution episcopic image (1352×1795 pixels, three colors) was taken before each slicing step; cf. Fig. 1(c) and Fig. 2(c).

Fig. 1(b) also displays a tissue slice after sectioning. The tissue slice was then stretched in warm water at 55°C for flattening. Thereafter, it was transferred onto a microscopic slide and dried. After drying, the sections were deparaffinized, stained in gallocyanin chromalum, and mounted under cover-glasses.

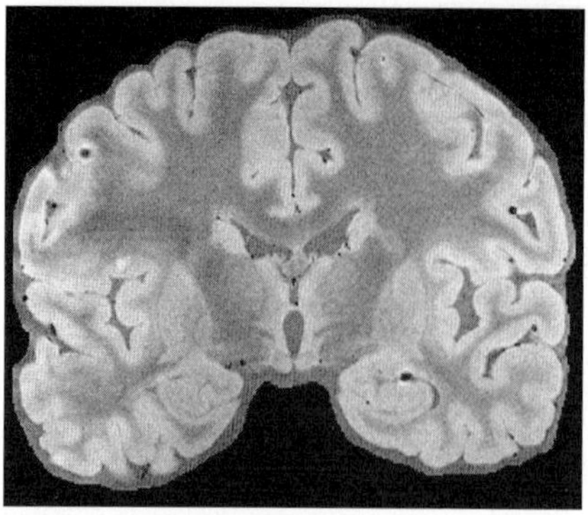

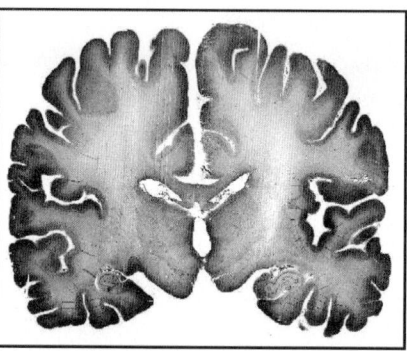

(a) slice of MRI scan

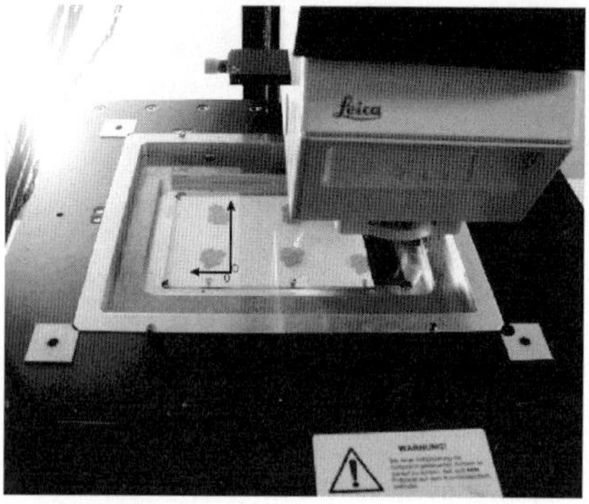

(b) light microscope

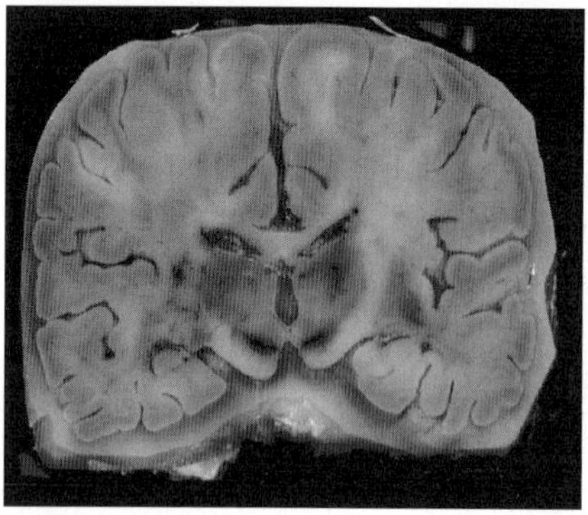

(c) episcope image

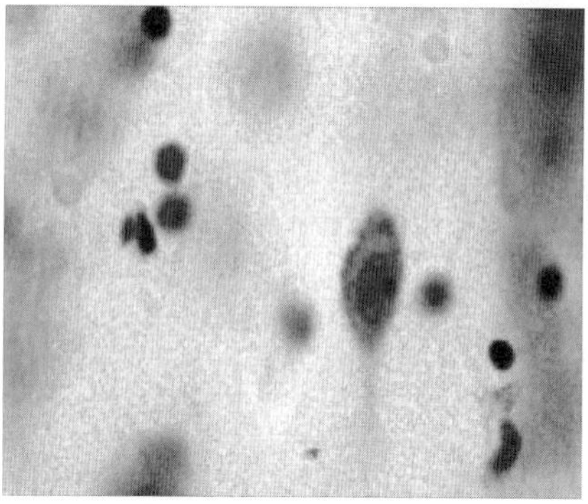

(d) cells

(e) scan of histological section

Fig. 2. Different image modalities of the brain: (a) MRI slice, (c) episcope image, (e) transparent flat bed scan of a microscopic slide; (b) light-microscope with microscopic slides on the table; (d) view through the microscope.

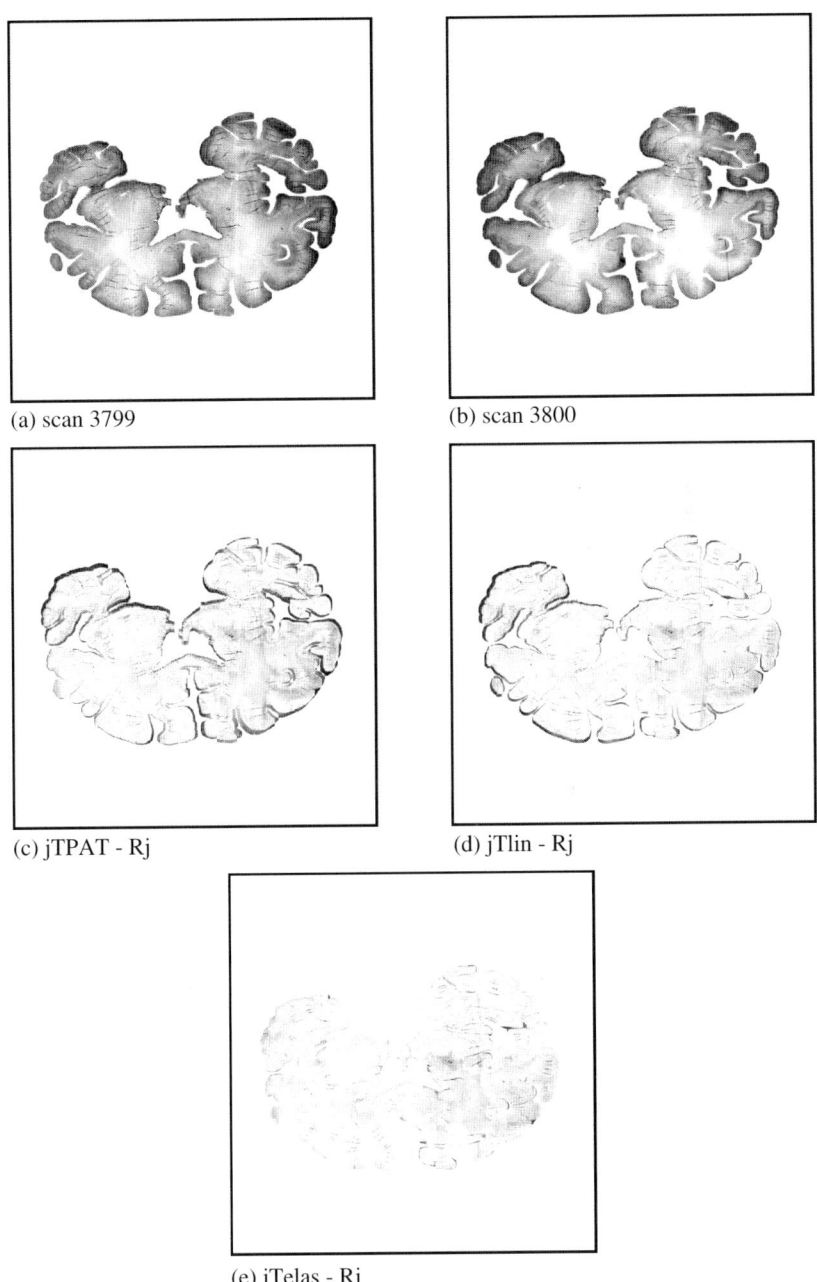

Fig. 3. Two consecutive axial scans 3799 (a) and 3800 (b) as well as difference images: (c) after PAT registration, (d) after optimal affine linear registration, and (e) after elastic registration.

A specialized light microscope with an extraordinarily large object range of 250×250 mm^2 is used to visualize all cells of the large tissue sections (Fig. 2(b,d)). Different neuronal entities were analyzed on different structural scales, i.e. from macroscopic details down to the cellular level; see [23] for the image processing. Although scanner technology has been improved tremendously within the last years, yet light-microscopy represents the only possibility to visualize fine details, like, for example, the exact spatial location of cells (Fig. 2(d)); cf. [23].

In order to relate the microscopic data to a macroscopic view of the slice and to recover the geometrical deformation of the tissue introduced by the various sectioning steps, flat bed scans of the slices were produced (Fig. 1(d) and Fig. 2(e)). These scans form the basis for our numerical treatment. Note, the fixed and mounted tissue sections can not be deformed whereas the scans (i.e. the digital images of the sections) can. Using a resolution of 2032 parts per inch in an 8 Bit gray-scale mode the digitized images range between 5000×2000 and 11000×7000 pixels (about 196 MBytes storage for the largest scan).

3 Registration Procedures

In this section we describe our reconstruction procedure for a stack of n scans. We use a continuous image model which enables us to use fast numerical schemes like, for example, Gauss-Newton schemes.

In Section 3.1 we discuss the discretization and interpolation schemes. In Section 3.2 we describe our preprocessing. The main objective is a segmentation of the scan of the brain and a gray value homogenization. The latter is necessary because the staining of consecutive section shows large variations. Section 3.3 summarizes general remarks concerning the registration of a stack of preprocessed scans. The second phase of our reconstruction, which may also be viewed as a further preprocessing step, consists of an affine linear registration; cf. Section 3.4. Here, the transformation can be phrased in terms of a small number of parameters and we end up with a parametric registration problem. The third and final phase consists of an elastic registration; cf. Section 3.5. For the affine linear and elastic registration we exploit a multilevel approach; see also [13, 14]. Here, the smoothed images are down-sampled and registration results obtained on a coarse level are used as starting values for the registration on the next finer level.

3.1 Discretization

Though the scans of the sections present discrete data, we prefer a continuous image model. Using a continuous model, the numerical schemes become independent of the actual image resolution and, most importantly, we are able to apply fast optimization schemes which typically rely on at least first order derivatives. However, for two reasons we ignore the need of differentiability of the transformed images and use a bilinear interpolation scheme, only. One reason is that higher order interpolation schemes, like, e.g. B-spline interpolations lead to oscillations and Gibbs phenomenon which are very pronounced at the cerebral cortex, of course. The second reason is that our numerical experiments strongly indicates that the benefit of higher order interpolation is hardly noticeable but the price in terms of computing time is quite high.

We assume all discrete data to be of the size m-by-n. The images are interpolated at pixel values (i, j) which are associated to points $(i/(m+1), j/(n+1)) \in \Omega :=]0, 1[^2$. For an arbitrary point (x, y) we set $T(x, y) = b$, if $(x, y) \notin \Omega$. Here, b is the gray value of the background which is typically zero. For the evaluation of $T(x, y)$, where $(x, y) \in \Omega$, we use a bilinear interpolation scheme based on the four closest pixels. Spatial derivatives are computed using central differences of the pre-smoothed image, where a convolution with a discrete Gaussian kernel is used for smoothing. For the computation of the two-dimensional integrals we use the midpoint quadrature rule.

3.2 Preprocessing

The stack of scans $S^{(j)}$, $j = 1, \ldots, n$, forms the basis for our numerical treatment. In a preprocessing step, each image is segmented using a simple but robust threshold based algorithm and it can be normalized using a PAT; cf., e.g., [1, 17].

Fig. 4 illustrates the normalization procedure for scan $S^{(3800)}$ of a human brain. The solid and dashed lines illustrate the first and second principal axis, respectively. The cross point is the center of gravity and the lengthes of the lines indicate the standard deviations in the principal directions. Note that the PAT registration is redundant. Moreover, particularly for scans resulting from corrupted sections, we observed that a PAT normalization can lead to an inferior starting point.

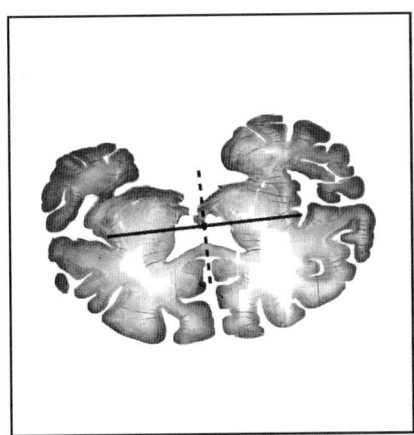 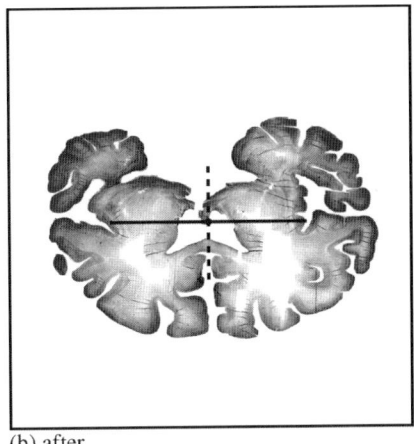

(a) before (b) after

Fig. 4. Scan before (a) and after (b) pre-registration. The solid and dashed lines illustrate the first and second principal axis, respectively. The cross point is the center of gravity and the lengthes indicate the standard deviations in principal directions.

Before registration we apply a gray value homogenization. We use the gray value statistic to equalize the gray value variation of the image stack which are due to staining variations. Let γ and σ denote the mean gray value and its standard deviation with respect to the non-zero image, respectively. With $\hat{\gamma}$ and $\hat{\sigma}$ we denote the target values obtained from a sliding median filtering of the corresponding values of the image stack. We replace the image S by $\hat{S} := \frac{\hat{\sigma}}{\sigma}(S - \gamma) + \hat{\gamma}$, where clipping is applied to out of range values. Hence, by linearity of the expectation value we have

$$\mathbb{E}[\hat{S}] = \frac{\hat{\sigma}}{\sigma}\mathbb{E}[S - \gamma] + \hat{\gamma} = \hat{\gamma} \quad \text{and} \quad \mathbb{E}[(\hat{S} - \hat{\gamma})^2] = \left(\frac{\hat{\sigma}}{\sigma}\right)^2 \mathbb{E}[(S - \gamma)^2] = \hat{\sigma}^2.$$

To minimize notational overhead, we subsequently denote the normalized scans also by $S^{(j)}$.

3.3 Stack Registration

Our registration is based on the L_2-difference or Sum of Squared Differences (SSD) (cf., e.g., [6])

$$D(A, B) := \frac{1}{2} \int_\Omega (A(x) - B(x))^2 \, d\mathbf{x}, \tag{1}$$

where A, B are two given images. For any image $S^{(j)}$ we consider an individual transformation $\mathbf{u}^{(j)}$, such that the joint distance

$$J(\mathbf{u}^{(1)}, \ldots, \mathbf{u}^{(n)}) := \sum_{j=2}^{n} D(S^{(j-1)} \circ \mathbf{u}^{(j-1)}, S^{(j)} \circ \mathbf{u}^{(j)})$$

$$= \frac{1}{2} \sum_{j=2}^{n} \int_\Omega \left(S^{(j-1)} \circ \mathbf{u}^{(j-1)} - S^{(j)} \circ \mathbf{u}^{(j)}\right)^2 dx \tag{2}$$

becomes minimal, where $(S^{(j)} \circ \mathbf{u}^{(j)})(\mathbf{x}) := S^{(j)}(\mathbf{u}^{(j)}(\mathbf{x}))$ denotes the transformed scan.

In order to avoid systematic scaling errors in the registration of the stack, the image $S^{(\nu)}$ with largest number of non-zero pixels remains unaltered throughout the registration, i.e. $\mathbf{u}^{(\nu)}(\mathbf{x}) = \mathbf{x}$. Therefore, the above minimization problem (2) decouples into two parts. Moreover, for the linear registration part, we constrain the transformations $\mathbf{u}^{(e)}$, $e = 1, n$, to be volume preserving, i.e.,

$$\det \nabla \mathbf{u}^{(e)} = 1. \tag{3}$$

Since a re-scaling of the images $S^{(e)}$ is already penalized by the elastic regularizer, we do not constrain $\mathbf{u}^{(e)}$ in the non-linear registration.

The constraints on $\mathbf{u}^{(e)}$ to be volume preserving is crucial, particularly when registering cone shaped objects. Without these additional constraints, one may obtains a cylinder shaped result. However, not all shape problems can be cured by this

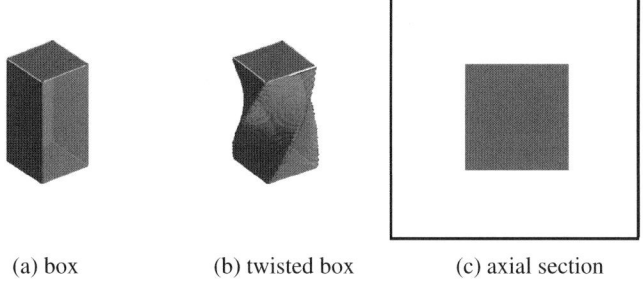

(a) box   (b) twisted box   (c) axial section

Fig. 5. Two three-dimensional objects, a box (a) and a twisted copy (b); arbitrary non-empty axial section through either of the two objects (c).

approach. Fig. 5 displays two three dimensional objects, a box and a twisted copy. If we would produce axial serial sectioning, we would obtain the same images for both objects; cf. Fig. 5(c). Therefore one has to face ambiguity in the reconstruction of three-dimensional objects from two-dimensional slices.

It is important to note that the registration discussed here aims to recover fine level details. Registration can not compensate for global shape variations, which are already introduced by removing the brain from the skull or by putting it onto a table. In order to correct for these global shape deformations, additional information has to be supplied. We will use an a priori taken magnetic resonance scan (MRI) of the brain (Fig. 2(a)) as a non-deformed reference and finally register our reconstruction to the MRI.

In the above discussion we assumed that the scan with maximal number of non-zero pixels is uniquely defined. However, the approach can be extended easily to the case when more than one scan take the maximum. As a matter of fact, we never observed this situation in our numerical experiments.

For the numerical minimization of J in (2), we use an iterative multilevel non-linear block Gauss-Seidel scheme. The iteration counter is denoted by k. For $k = 0$, we set $\mathbf{u}_k^{(j)}$ such that the associated map becomes the identity, $\mathbf{u}_k^{(j)}(\mathbf{x}) = \mathbf{x}$, $j = 1, \ldots, n$. For $j = 1, \ldots, n$, $j \neq \nu$, we minimize

$$\hat{J}_j(\mathbf{u}^{(j)}) := J(\mathbf{u}_{k+1}^{(1)}, \ldots, \mathbf{u}_{k+1}^{(j-1)}, \mathbf{u}^{(j)}, \mathbf{u}_k^{(j+1)}, \ldots, \mathbf{u}_k^{(n)}), \quad (4)$$

with respect to $\mathbf{u}^{(j)}$ only and the minimizer is denoted by $\mathbf{u}_{k+1}^{(j)}$. Setting $k \mapsto k + 1$ we repeat the iteration until stagnation in the distance measure J is observed.

Of course, other optimization strategies can be used as well. However, a discussion is beyond the scope of this paper and we therefore refer to the optimization literature; see, e.g., [18] and references therein.

Note that the minimization in (4) is only with respect to $\mathbf{u}^{(j)}$. With $\hat{S}_k^{(j)}$ denoting the deformed image, $\hat{S}_k^{(j)}(\mathbf{x}) = S^{(j)}(\mathbf{u}_k^{(j)}(\mathbf{x}))$ and some constants d we have

$$\hat{J}_1(\mathbf{u}^{(1)}) = D(S^{(1)} \circ \mathbf{u}^{(1)}, \hat{S}_k^{(2)}) + d,$$

$$\hat{J}_n(\mathbf{u}^{(n)}) = D(S^{(n)} \circ \mathbf{u}^{(n)}, \hat{S}_k^{(n-1)}) + d,$$

$$\hat{J}_j(\mathbf{u}^{(j)}) = D(\hat{S}_{k+1}^{(j-1)}, S^{(j)} \circ \mathbf{u}^{(j)}) + D(S^{(j)} \circ \mathbf{u}^{(j)}, \hat{S}_k^{(j+1)}) + d_1$$

$$= D(S^{(j)} \circ \mathbf{u}^{(j)}, \frac{1}{2}\hat{S}_{k+1}^{(j-1)} + \frac{1}{2}\hat{S}_k^{(j+1)}) + d_2.$$

Therefore, a minimizer of (4) can be obtained by minimizing

$$J_2(\mathbf{u}) := D(R, T \circ \mathbf{u}), \tag{5}$$

where

$$T := S^{(j)} \quad \text{and} \quad R := \begin{cases} \frac{1}{2}(\hat{S}_{k+1}^{(j-1)} + \hat{S}_k^{(j+1)}), & 1 < j < n, \\ \hat{S}_k^{(2)}, & j = 1, \\ \hat{S}_k^{(n-1)}, & j = n. \end{cases}$$

As already pointed out, we apply a multilevel approach for the minimization of (5). The images on the fine grid are smoothed by convolving with a discrete Gaussian kernel and are down-sampled to a coarse grid. The registration results on the coarse grid are mapped to the fine grid and serve as generally excellent starting values for the registration on the fine grid.

3.4 Affine Linear Registration

Since an affine linear transformation $\mathbf{u}$ belongs to a finite dimensional space, it can be parameterized like, for example,

$$\mathbf{u}(\mathbf{x}) := \begin{pmatrix} u_1 x_1 + u_2 x_2 + u_3 \\ u_4 x_1 + u_5 x_2 + u_6 \end{pmatrix} \tag{6}$$

and we therefore associate $\mathbf{u}$ with the parameter vector $(u_1, \ldots, u_6)$. For the volume preserving map we use the parameterization

$$\mathbf{u}^{(e)}(\mathbf{x}) = \begin{pmatrix} 1 & u_1^{(e)} \\ 0 & 1 \end{pmatrix} \begin{pmatrix} \cos u_2^{(e)} & -\sin u_2^{(e)} \\ \sin u_2^{(e)} & \cos u_2^{(e)} \end{pmatrix} \begin{pmatrix} x_1 \\ x_2 \end{pmatrix} + \begin{pmatrix} u_3^{(e)} \\ u_4^{(e)} \end{pmatrix},$$

where the first matrix describes shear and the second rotation.

For a numerical solution of (5) we exploit a Gauss-Newton scheme, where only first order derivatives of the images are needed; cf., e.g., [18]. Starting with an initial guess $\mathbf{u}_0$, we obtain $\mathbf{u}_{k+1} = \mathbf{u}_k + \delta\mathbf{u}$, where $\delta\mathbf{u}$ is the solution of the linearized L_2 approximation problem

$$\|R - T \circ \mathbf{u}_{k+1}\| \approx \|R - T \circ \mathbf{u}_k - \nabla_\mathbf{u}[T \circ \mathbf{u}]_{\mathbf{u}=\mathbf{u}_k} \delta\mathbf{u}\| = \min.$$

The generic derivative $\nabla_{\mathbf{u}}[T \circ \mathbf{u}]$ is given by

$$\partial_{u_1}[T \circ \mathbf{u}] = \partial_1 T \cdot x_1, \quad \partial_{u_4}[T \circ \mathbf{u}] = \partial_2 T \cdot x_1,$$
$$\partial_{u_2}[T \circ \mathbf{u}] = \partial_1 T \cdot x_2, \quad \partial_{u_5}[T \circ \mathbf{u}] = \partial_2 T \cdot x_2,$$
$$\partial_{u_3}[T \circ \mathbf{u}] = \partial_1 T, \quad \partial_{u_6}[T \circ \mathbf{u}] = \partial_2 T,$$

where the directional derivatives $\partial_j T = \partial_j T(\mathbf{u}(\mathbf{x}))$ are approximated by centered finite difference approximation of the smoothed images T; cf. Section 3.1. The derivatives for the first and last section are given by

$$\partial_{u_1^{(e)}}[T \circ \mathbf{u}^{(e)}] = \partial_1 T \cdot (sx_1 + cx_2),$$
$$\partial_{u_2^{(e)}}[T \circ \mathbf{u}^{(e)}] = \partial_1 T \cdot ((ca - s)x_1 - (c + as)x_2) - \partial_2 T(-cx_1 + sx_2),$$
$$\partial_{u_3^{(e)}}[T \circ \mathbf{u}^{(e)}] = \partial_1 T,$$
$$\partial_{u_4^{(e)}}[T \circ \mathbf{u}^{(e)}] = \partial_2 T.$$

3.5 Elastic Registration

As it is apparent from Fig. 3(d), an affine linear registration alone does not lead to satisfying reconstruction results. Therefore, a non-linear registration becomes necessary. Here, we use an elastic registration which has been studied for over 20 years; see, e.g., [5, 3, 7, 10, 17].

The basic idea of elastic registration can be described as follows. Assume that the template image has been painted onto a rubber. A deformation of the rubber results in a deformed template image but also introduces a potential energy to the rubber. The stronger the deformation the higher this potential becomes. The idea is to find a deformation which minimizes both, the distance between reference and deformed template as well as the elastic potential. Therefore, deformations leading to a very high elastic potential become disregarded even if they lead to small values of D. In other words, the distance measure (5) is regularized by the elastic potential and the registration problem becomes

$$J_{elas}(\mathbf{u}) = D(R, T \circ \mathbf{u}) + S(\mathbf{u}) = \min, \tag{7}$$

where

$$S(\mathbf{u}) = \int_{\mathbb{R}^2} \frac{\lambda}{2}(\operatorname{div} \mathbf{u})^2 + \mu\left\{(\partial_1 u_1)^2 + (\partial_2 u_2)^2 + \frac{1}{2}(\partial_1 u_2 + \partial_2 u_1)^2\right\} dx \tag{8}$$

and μ and λ are the so-called Lamé constants reflecting material properties; see, e.g., [17] for details.

This particular regularization in our registration scheme is motivated by the fact that the histological sections originally consist of almost pure paraffin wax. The deformation process due to sectioning is therefore expected to be dominated by the elastic properties of the section. Note that also other processes like, e.g., drying or mounting contributes to the overall deformations.

Note that in contrast to the affine linear registration where **u** is described in terms of at most six parameters, the deformation in the continuous formulation of the nonlinear registration is not restricted to a finite dimensional search space. However, in our implementation we use a discretization where values of **u**(**x**) are computed for each pixel **x**.

Following [9], a minimizer is characterized by the Euler-Lagrange equations

$$\mathcal{A}\mathbf{u}(\mathbf{x}) + \mathbf{f}(\mathbf{x}, \mathbf{u}(\mathbf{x})) = 0 \quad \text{for all} \quad \mathbf{x} \in \Omega, \tag{9}$$

where the well-known Navier-Lamé operator $\mathcal{A}$ is related to the Gâteaux-derivative of $\mathcal{S}$,

$$\mathcal{A}[\mathbf{u}] = \mu \Delta \mathbf{u} + (\lambda + \mu) \nabla \operatorname{div} \mathbf{u}$$
$$= \mu \begin{pmatrix} \partial_{1,1} u_1 + \partial_{2,2} u_1 \\ \partial_{1,1} u_2 + \partial_{2,2} u_2 \end{pmatrix} + (\lambda + \mu) \begin{pmatrix} \partial_{1,1} u_1 \partial_{1,2} + u_2 \\ \partial_{1,2} u_1 \partial_{2,2} + u_2 \end{pmatrix}$$

and the so-called force **f** is related to the Gâteaux-derivative of $\mathcal{D}$,

$$\mathbf{f}(\mathbf{x}, \mathbf{u}(\mathbf{x})) = \Big(R(\mathbf{x}) - T(\mathbf{x} + \mathbf{u}(\mathbf{x})) \Big) \cdot \nabla T(\mathbf{x} + \mathbf{u}(\mathbf{x})). \tag{10}$$

For the computation of a numerical solution, we used the scheme proposed in [9].

4 Results

Fig. 6 displays some results for the registration of a stack of $n = 503$ slices from a *Sprague Dawley* rat brain. Each scan has a resolution of 1900×1900 pixels, which ends up in a total amount of 1.7 gigabytes (GB) of data. Heavily corrupted tissue sections were automatically detected and disregarded, such that 474 scans (1.6 GB) remained.

Fig. 6(a) displays a view of the non-registered stack and (b) a view of the elastically registered stack. To illustrate the value of the reconstruction, we resampled the data orthogonally to the direction of sectioning and show a virtual sagittal slice; see Fig. 7.

In the virtual sagittal slice structures like, for example, the cerebellar fissures, molecular and granular layer, and white substance of cerebellum are clearly recognizable. Note that the initial fuzzy looking brain now offers morphological details and obviously dramatic increase of surface smoothness. Overall, the displaced areas are coherent again. It should be noted, that the registration is an indispensable technique for recognition, discussion and three-dimensional measurement of internal and external morphologic entities.

For this reconstruction, a linear pre-registration based on the principle axis transformation was performed. The error (cf. (2)) decreased by about 27%, i.e.

$$J(\mathbf{u}_{\text{PAT}}) \approx 0.73 \cdot J(\mathbf{u}_0).$$

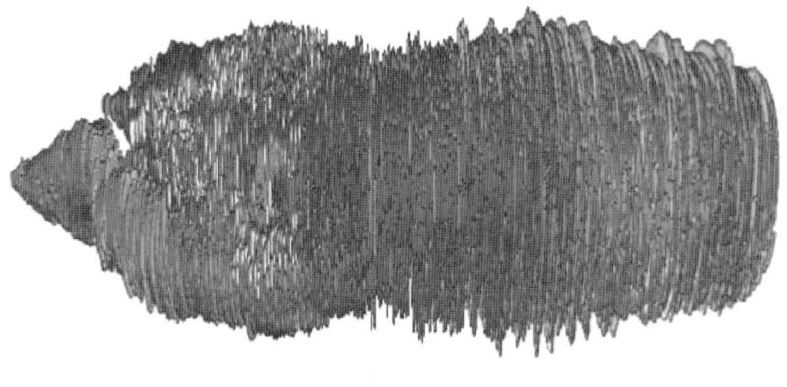

(a) no registration

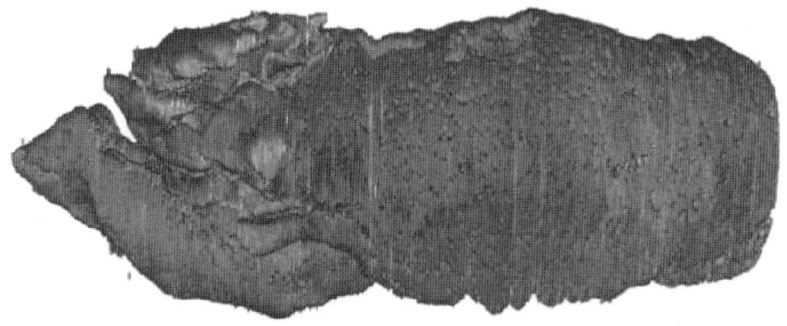

(b) elastic registration

Fig. 6. Lateral view of the three-dimensional reconstruction of a whole rat brain; (a) no registration and (b) elastic registration.

For this reconstruction, it turned out that a pure elastic registration through five levels of a Gaussian pyramid (coarsest images 128×128 pixels) leads to a satisfying convergence. No PAT pre-registration was applied. The MATLAB [15] implemented registration algorithm lasted about ten hours for the high-resolution images on a AMD Athlon XP 2700+, 1GB RAM, running Linux.

Only 35 iteration steps were needed and the error decreased by 79%, i.e.

$$J(\mathbf{u}_{elas}) \approx 0.21 \cdot J(\mathbf{u}_0).$$

In Tab. 1 the runtime results for the registration of images in different resolutions is assembled.

Beside measuring the registration results with the distance measure $\mathcal{D}$, the results were evaluated by an anatomist. An important criterium is the improvement

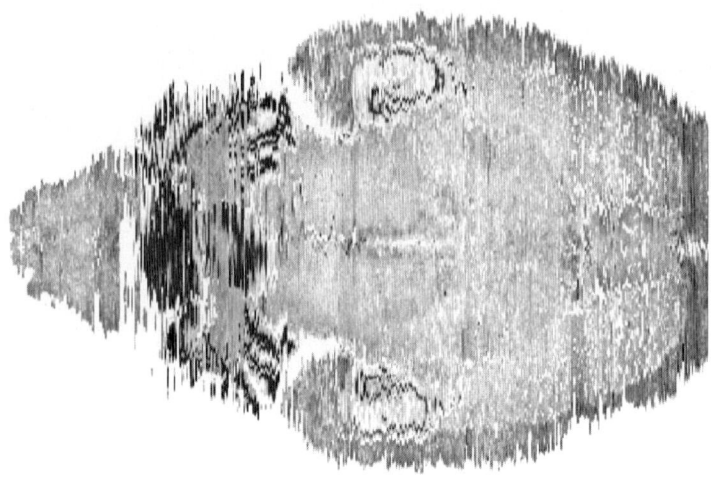

(a) no registration

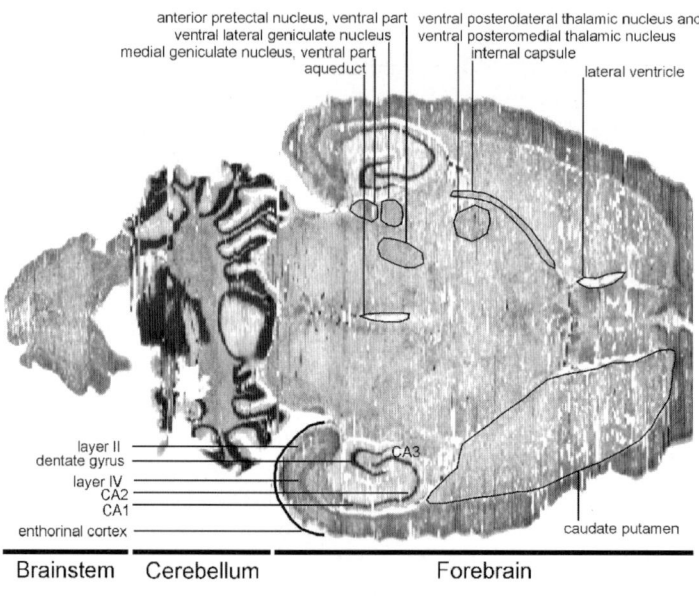

(b) elastic registration

Fig. 7. Reproduced virtual slice (sagittal, orthogonal to the sectioning direction, Bregma -5.82 mm, Interaural 4.18 mm; see, e.g., Paxinos & Watson [20]). A column of the virtual slice represents the intersection of the virtual slice with an original slice (axial); (a) no registration, (b) after elastic registration. Note that registration enables the identification of anatomical structure.

Table 1. Computational costs of the registration versus data dimensions; MB gives the storage requirements of the data, #levels the number of levels used in our multiscale approach, t_{iter} is the CPU time in minutes needed for one iteration on the finest grid, t_{total} is the total CPU time needed for the registration, and #iter is the overall number of iterations on all levels. The whole reconstruction process takes about ten hours CPU time using MATLAB [15] on a AMD Athlon XP 2700+, 1GB RAM, running Linux.

data dimensions	MB	#levels	t_{iter} (min)	t_{total} (min)	#iter
$128 \times 128 \times 474$	8	1	0.5	9	19
$256 \times 256 \times 474$	30	2	1.9	32	24
$512 \times 512 \times 474$	119	3	10.7	125	28
$1024 \times 1024 \times 474$	474	4	42.9	240	32
$1900 \times 1900 \times 474$	1632	5	149.5	547	35

of the representation of small structures (subcortical nuclei, cortical areas) and the smoothness of inner and outer borders. The registered slices do fulfill this requirement. Generally, three classes of neuroanatomical structures are recognizable only after registration: 1) subcortical nuclei, 2) ventricles, and 3) certain cerebral and cerebellar cytoarchitectonic layers. More precisely, subcortical nuclei like the caudate putamen complex, medial geniculate nucleus - ventral part, anterior pretectal nucleus - ventral part, ventral posterolateral thalamic nucleus, ventral posteromedial thalamic nucleus among other things can be localized. Furthermore, the lateral ventricle and the aqueduct become visible. Finally, cytoarchitectonic layering at certain parts of the cerebral and the cerebellar cortex can be detected. In the forebrain one can observe hippocampal substructures like the CA1, CA2, CA3 regions (CA: cornu amonis) and the dentate gyrus, see Fig. 7. Moreover, in the entorhinal region the layer II (external granular layer) and IV (internal granular layer) are distinguishable.

In Fig. 8 the results of the registration processes are visualized in detail for a part of the rat brain. Fig. 8 depicts the three-dimensional reconstruction of 68 slices before (a) and after (b) registration. The massively shifted images yield to an blurred reconstruction without recognizable fine anatomic details (Fig. 8(c)). Fig. 8 also illustrates the variation of the internal structures before (c) and after (d) registration by means of virtual slice orthogonal to the sectioning direction. Note, that the registration results allows for a detailed discussion of the internal structures.

5 Conclusions

We presented the first fully reconstructed rat brain at a resolution at level of the micrometer scale. The huge amount of data (≈ 1.6 GB) as well as the required quality demand for a special registration technique. Only the use of a specific variational technique accompanied by strategies to incorporate special properties of the underlying tissue enables us to match the high anatomical demands.

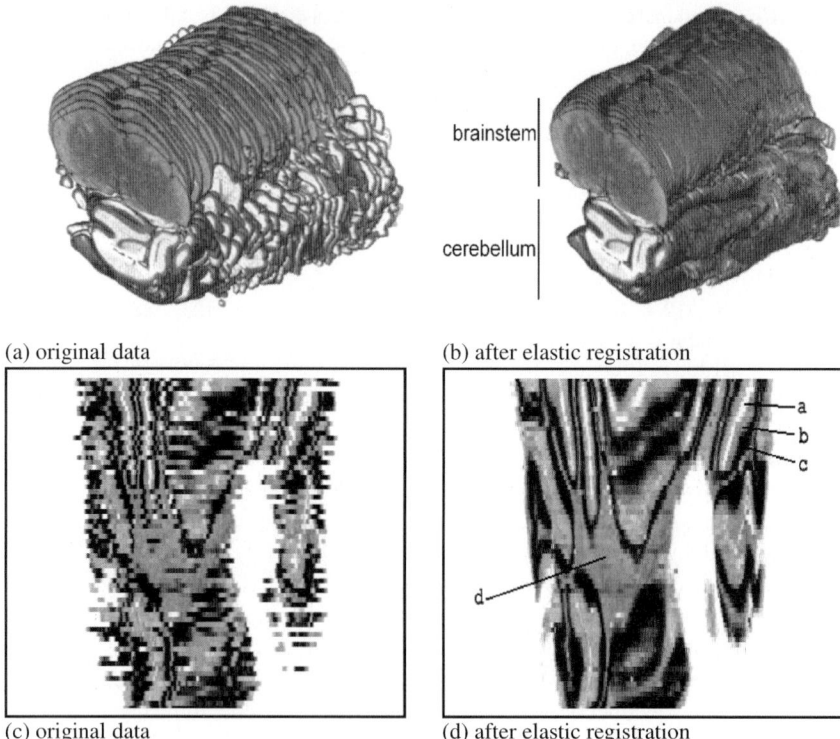

Fig. 8. Three-dimensional lateral view of a part of the rat brain and virtual orthogonal slices; (a) original data, (b) after elastic registration. This part of the brain shows the brainstem at the top and the cerebellum with folia at the bottom. The virtual slices (orthogonal to the sectioning direction) demonstrate the morphologic effect of registration: (c) original data, (d) after elastic registration. Recognizable structures after registration: a cerebellar fissures, b molecular layer, c granular layer, d white substance of the cerebellum.

The backbone of the scheme is a super-fast solution technique for the inner linear system. This technique is accompanied by sound strategies for accelerating the outer iteration. This includes a multi-scale approach based on a Gaussian pyramid as well as a sophisticated estimation of the material constants for the elastic potential.

The results of the registration process enable the identification of histological details that pertain to three distinct groups of neuroanatomical structures: subcortical nuclei, ventricles and cerebellar or cerebral cytoarchitectonic layers. Before registration the detection of these structures was impossible. Therefore, it is essential to apply elastic registration to this kind of non-linear problem. Furthermore, now it is feasible to develop strategies for three-dimensional morphometric analysis of specific areas in registered stacks of images derived from normal and pathologic brains for experimental studies. Finally, the obvious advantages were quantified by a distance measure leading to an improvement of about 79% after just 35 iteration steps.

Currently we are working at a full reconstruction of a human brain. Here the task is to align about 6000 slices of dimension (12000 × 7000) pixels (resolution: 31.75μm per pixel)! Preliminary results look very promising and indicate that the outlined approach is capable of dealing with such an amount of data on a PC from the shelf.

References

1. N. M. Alpert, J. F. Bradshaw, D. Kennedy and J. A. Correia: The principal axes transformation – A method for image registration, Journal of nuclear medicine **31/10**, pp 1717-1722, (1990)
2. V. Arsigny, X. Pennec and N. Ayache: A novel family of geometrical transformations: Polyrigid transformations. application to the registration of histological slices, Research report 4837, INRIA, (2003)
3. R. Bajcsy and S. Kovačič: Toward an individualized brain atlas elastic matching, Tech. Report MS-CIS-86-71 Grasp Lap 76, Dept. of Computer and Information Science, Moore School, University of Philadelphia, (1986)
4. H. Benveniste and S. Blackland: MR microscopy and high resolution small animal MRI: applications in neuroscience research, Progress in Neurobiology, **67**, pp 393-420, (2002)
5. C. Broit: Optimal registration of deformed images, Ph.D. thesis, Computer and Information Science, University of Pensylvania, (1981)
6. L. G. Brown: A survey of image registration techniques, ACM Computing Surveys, **24/4**, pp 325-376, (1992)
7. G. E. Christensen: Deformable shape models for anatomy, Ph.D. thesis, Sever Institute of Technology, Washington University, (1994)
8. T. Delzescaux, J. Dauguet, F. Condé, R. Maroy and V. Frouin: Using 3d non rigid FFD-based method to register post mortem 3d histological data and in vivo MRI of a baboon brain, MICCAI 2003 (R. E. Ellis and T. M. Peters (Eds.), LNCS, Springer, **2879**, pp 965-966, (2003)
9. B. Fischer and J. Modersitzki: Fast inversion of matrices arising in image processing, Num. Algo. **22**, pp 1-11 (1999)
10. J. C. Gee, D. R. Haynor, L. Le Briquer and R. Bajcsy: Advances in elastic matching theory and its implementation, CVRMed, pp 63-72, (1997)
11. S. C. Grant, D. L. Buckley, S. Gibbs, A. G. Web and S. J. Blackland: MR microscopy of multicomponent diffusion in single neurons, Magnetic Resonance in Medicine **46**, pp 1107-1112, (2001)
12. S. Henn and K. Witsch: Iterative multigrid regularization techniques for image matching, SIAM J. on Scientific Comp. **23/4**, pp 1077-1093, (2001)
13. B. Jähne: Digital image processing, 4th ed., Springer, (1997)
14. J. Kybic and M. Unser: Multidimensional elastic registration of images using splines, ICIP in Vancouver, 10.-13.09.2000, pp 1-4, (September 2000)
15. MathWorks, Natick, Mass.: Matlab user's guide, (1992)
16. C. R. Maurer and J. M. Fitzpatrick: Interactive image-guided neurosurgery, ch. A Review of Medical Image Registration, pp. 17-44, Park Ridge, IL, American Association of Neurological Surgeons, (1993)

17. J. Modersitzki: Numerical methods for image registration, Oxford University Press, (2004)
18. J. Nocedal and S. J. Wright: Numerical optimization, Springer, New York (1999)
19. S. Ourselin, A. Roche, G. Subsol, X. Pennec and C. Sattonnet: Automatic alignment of histological sections for 3D reconstruction and analysis, Tech. Report 3595, Institut National de Recherche en Informatique et en Automatique, France, (Dec. 1998)
20. G. Paxinos C. and Watson: The rat brain in stereotaxic coordinates, 4th ed., Academic Press, (1998)
21. A. Pitiot, G. Malandain, E. Bardinet and P. Thompson: Piecewise Affine Registration of Biological Images, WBIR 2003 (Gee, J.C. and Maintz, J.B.A. and Vannier, M.W. - Eds.), LNCS, **2717**, Springer, pp 91-101, (2003)
22. K. Rohr: Landmark-based image analysis, Computational Imaging and Vision, Kluwer Academic Publishers, Dordrecht, (2001)
23. O. Schmitt: Die multimodale Architektonik des menschlichen Gehirns, Habilitation, Insitute of Anatomy, Medical University of Lübeck, Germany, (2001)
24. A. W. Toga and J. C. Mazziotta: Brain mapping: The methods, 2nd ed., Academic Press, (2002)

Computational Methods for Nonlinear Image Registration

Ulrich Clarenz[1], Marc Droske[2], Stefan Henn[3], Martin Rumpf[4], and Kristian Witsch[5]

[1] Institut für Mathematik, Gerhard-Mercator Universität Duisburg, Lotharstraße 63/65, 47048 Duisburg, Germany.
 clarenz@math.uni-duisburg.de
[2] Math Sciences Department, University of California, 520 Portola Plaza, Los Angeles, CA, 90055, USA.
 droske@math.ucla.edu
[3] Lehrstuhl für Mathematische Optimierung, Mathematisches Institut, Heinrich-Heine Universität Düsseldorf, Universitätsstraße 1, D-40225 Düsseldorf, Germany.
 henn@am.uni-duesseldorf.de
[4] Institut für Numerische Simulation, Rheinische Friedrich-Wilhelms-Universität Bonn, Nussallee 15, D-53115 Bonn, Germany.
 martin.rumpf@ins.uni-bonn.de
[5] Lehrstuhl für Angewandte Mathematik, Mathematisches Institut, Heinrich-Heine Universität Düsseldorf, Universitätsstraße 1, D-40225 Düsseldorf, Germany.
 witsch@am.uni-duesseldorf.de

Summary Image registration is the process of the alignment of two or more data sets recorded with the same or different imaging machineries. Especially nonlinear image registration techniques allow the alignment of data sets that are mismatched in a nonuniform manner. Mathematically, this yields a nonlinear ill–conditioned inverse problem. In this presentation, we introduce several computational methods based on variational PDE approaches to obtain an approximate solution of the nonlinear registration problem. In each approach we have to solve a sequence of subproblems. Each subproblem has to be well-posed and should be efficiently solvable.

1 Introduction

The following contribution gives an overview on variational techniques which are used to solve the so called image matching or template matching problem. The origin of this problem is in medical applications, especially image assisted diagnostics and surgery planning. Here, physicians often need robust and valid segmentation and classification results as well as an analysis of the temporal change of anatomic structures. To this aim they want to correlate images recorded with different imaging machinery or at different times in a suitable way. There is a rich theory and also a large number of algorithms to to solve this registration problem. They all ask for an "optimal" deformation which deforms one image such that there is an "optimal" correlation to another image with respect to a suitable coherence or difference measure. The pure minimization of such difference measures typically leads to an ill-posed problem (see section 3). Therefore regularization approaches must be taken into account.

Mainly two different regularization techniques have been discussed in the literature [5, 6, 10, 15, 23, 25, 32]. On the one hand, so called elastic registration techniques deal with a regularization of the energy, typically adding a convex energy functional based on gradients to the actual matching energy. The regularization energy is regarded as a penalty for "elastic stresses" resulting from the deformation of the images. This approach is related to the well known classical Tikhonov regularization of the originally ill-posed problem. On the other hand, viscous flow techniques are taken into account. They compute smooth paths from some initial deformation towards the set of minimizers of the matching energy. Thereby, a suitable regularization of the velocity, e.g., adding an artificial viscosity, ensures a certain problem dependent smoothness modulus. This class of methods can be interpreted as a gradient flow approach with respect to a metric which penalizes non–regular descent directions. Taking into account a time-step discretization this methodology is closely related to iterative Tikhonov regularization methods [16, 31, 18].

A mixture of these approaches is used in [12], where on the one hand an elastic energy is added to the difference measure, on the other hand a regularized gradient flow is taken into account.

The aim of this contribution is to give a systematic overview on all these techniques, i.e., dealing with a similarity measure leading to an ill-posed problem and the corresponding regularization aspects.

In section 2 we discuss the general nature of image matching in more detail. Especially, we will show that variational approaches are a natural way to solve those matching problems section 2.2. In section 3 we will explain why using only the difference measures leads to ill-posed problems. The corresponding regularization aspects are discussed in section 4. An overview of possible combinations of matching energies and regularizations is given in section 5. Note that the non–convexity of the minimization problem in image registration makes it difficult to find the absolute minimum of a chosen matching energy in case of larger deformations. Alternatively, one can consider a convolution of the images with a large corresponding filter width which destroys much of the detailed structure, match those images, and then successively reduce the filter-width and iterate the process [2, 28, 35]. This kind of preconditioning is explained in section 5.5.

2 A Variational Formulation

Given two images $T, R : \Omega \to \mathbb{R}$, where $\Omega \subset \mathbb{R}^d$ and $d = 2, 3$, we would like to determine a deformation $\phi : \Omega \to \mathbb{R}^d$ which maps the first image T via a deformation ϕ to the second image R such that corresponding structures are mapped onto each other. In the following we call the image T the template and R the reference.

Many image analysis methodologies have been developed to tackle this problem. Image registration strategies are normally classified in two general categories.

On the one hand, there exist feature-based methods, i.e., the deformation is calculated based on a number of "anatomical" correspondences established manually, or automatically on a number of distinguish "anatomical" features, such as distinct landmark-point [29] or a combination of curves and surfaces, e.g. see [33]. On the other hand methods based on volumetric transformations are considered. This methods seek to maximize the similarity between the template and the reference via a deformation.

In many practical applications only a noisy version R^δ of the exact data R is given with

$$||R - R^\delta|| \leq \delta$$

with unknown noise level δ. We furthermore expect $\phi(\Omega) = \Omega$. For the ease of presentation we assume $\Omega = [0,1]^d$ throughout this paper. We consider u as the displacement corresponding to ϕ: $\mathbb{I} + u = \phi$.

In this section we want to collect examples of similarity measures. Here, a lot of choices are possible depending on the application one has in mind. At this point one may distinguish two fundamental cases:

2.1 Mono-modal Matching Energies

Let us start with the easier case of monomodal matching. Given are two (or more) images, where similar structures are represented by similar grey-values. In this case one usually aims for the deformation ϕ that

$$T \circ \phi \approx R.$$

The most basic energy D depending on the displacement u (resp. the deformation ϕ) is the L^2-distance:

$$D^{LSQ}[u] = \frac{1}{2} \int_\Omega |T \circ (\mathbb{I} + u) - R|^2 . \tag{D}$$

In what follows we use either ϕ or u as the argument of the energy D. If u is an ideal deformation the above energy vanishes. Thus we ask for solutions of the problem to minimize $D^{LSQ}[\cdot]$ for u in some Banach space $\mathcal{X}$.

A minimizer u of (6) is characterized by the necessary condition $(D^{LSQ})'[u] = 0$, where $(D^{LSQ})'[u] \in \mathcal{X}'$ for the dual space $\mathcal{X}'$ of $\mathcal{X}$. Indeed, we require

$$\langle (D^{LSQ})'[u], \varphi \rangle = 0 \quad \forall \varphi \in \mathcal{X} .$$

Suppose $[L^2(\Omega)]^d$ is embedded in the space $\mathcal{X}'$. Under certain regularity assumptions on T, R and ∇T we obtain the L^2-representation of $(D^{LSQ})'$

$$\mathrm{grad}_{L^2} D^{LSQ}[u] = (T \circ (\mathbb{I} + u) - R) \nabla T \circ (\mathbb{I} + u) . \tag{1}$$

In the following sections we will especially focus on this special choice of distance measure.

2.2 Multi-modal Matching Energies

In general, if the images are recorded with different imaging machinery, the so-called multi-modal registration, the D^{LSQ} functional is not an appropriate measure. The main reason is that the same structures may have quite different gray values in the multi-modal case. In this case the use of (D) does not make any sense.

Mutual Information Energy One frequently used approach to this problem is the so called mutual information strategy [14, 24, 34, 36]. There, one searches for an affine-linear transformation so that the mutual information (or transinformation) is maximized. Nonlinear approaches are presented, e.g in [9, 19, 21, 20]. Mutual information is borrowed from information theory, see e.g. [4]. The mutual information between two discrete random variables X and Y is defined to be

$$I(X,Y) = H(X) + H(Y) - H(X,Y),$$

where $H(X)$ is the entropy of the random variable X and $H(X,Y)$ is the joint entropy of these variables.

This intensity based matching energy was introduced in the context of multi-modal image-registration in [34]. Using our notation, the mutual-information based matching energy is defined by

$$D^{MI}[u] = I(T \circ (\mathbb{1} + u), R).$$

The mutual information based matching energy is maximal if the images are matched. Therefore the mutual information based matching energy is a measure of alignment between the images. This signifies that we have to maximize $D^{MI}[u]$ or equivalently minimize $D^{-MI}[u] := -D^{MI}[u]$. Confer to figure J or an example of an MRI-CT matching of the brain based on this similarity measure.

Morphological Matching Energy A disadvantage of the Mutual Information approach is its global character. Indeed our energy integral is an integral in the space of grey values where the corresponding energy density is nonlocal and consists of the probability distributions. We might ask for a local energy density reflecting solely the morphology. Thus, let us define the morphology $M[I]$ of an image I as the set of level sets of I:

$$M[I] := \{\mathcal{M}_c^I \mid c \in \mathbb{R}\},$$

where $\mathcal{M}_c^I := \{x \in \Omega \mid I(x) = c\}$ is a single level set for the grey value c. I.e. $M[\gamma \circ I] = M[I]$ for any reparametrization $\gamma : \mathbb{R} \to \mathbb{R}$ of the grey values. Up to the orientation the morphology $M[I]$ can be identified with the normal map (Gauss map)

$$N_I : \Omega \to \mathbb{R}^d \, ; \, x \mapsto \frac{\nabla I}{\|\nabla I\|}.$$

Morphological methods in image processing are characterized by an invariance with respect to the morphology [30]. Now, aiming for a morphological multi-modal registration method, we will ask for a deformation $\phi : \Omega \to \Omega$ such that

$$M[T \circ \phi] = M[R].$$

Thus, we set up a matching functional which locally measures the twist of the tangent spaces of the template image at the deformed position and the deformed reference image or the defect of the corresponding normal fields. We aim to minimize a suitable matching energy, which measures the morphological defect of the reference image R and the deformed template image T, i. e., we ask for a deformation ϕ such that $N_T \circ \phi || N_R^\phi$, where N_R^ϕ is the transformed normal of the reference image R on $T_{\phi(x)}\phi(\mathcal{M}_{R(x)}^R)$ at position $\phi(x)$. Here, $T_y\mathcal{M}$ denotes the tangent space of a surface $\mathcal{M}$ at a position y. From the transformation rule for the exterior vector product $D\phi\, u \wedge D\phi\, v = \text{cof} D\phi(u \wedge v)$ for all vectors v, w which are tangential to the level set $\mathcal{M}_{R(x)}^R$ one derives

$$N_R^\phi = \frac{\text{cof} D\phi\, N_R}{\|\text{cof} D\phi\, N_R\|}$$

where $\text{cof} A = \det A \cdot A^{-T}$ for invertible $A \in \mathbb{R}^{d,d}$ is the cofactor matrix of A - a matrix consisting of all $(n-1)$-minors of A. Thus, we have for $D\phi$:

$$n = 2 : \quad \text{cof} D\phi = \begin{bmatrix} \partial_2\phi_2 & -\partial_2\phi_1 \\ -\partial_1\phi_2 & \partial_1\phi_1 \end{bmatrix}$$

$$n = 3 : \quad (\text{cof} D\phi)_{ij} = \partial_{i+1}\phi_{i+1}\partial_{i+2}\phi_{i+2} - \partial_{i+1}\phi_{i+2}\partial_{i+2}\phi_{i+1}.$$

with cyclic indices. Now, one might be tempted to define the matching energy $\int_\Omega \|N_T \circ \phi - N_R^\phi\|^2 d\mu$. But, for a better treatment of the singularities [12], we avoid the normalization appearing in N_R^ϕ and choose the following matching energy

$$D^{morph}[\phi] := \int_\Omega g_0(\nabla T \circ \phi, \nabla R, cof D\phi) d\mu.$$

where g_0 is a 0-homogenous extension of a function $g : S^{d-1} \times S^{d-1} \times \mathbb{R}^{d,d} \to \mathbb{R}^+$, i. e., $g_0(v, w, A) := 0$ if $v = 0$ or $w = 0$ and $g_0(v, w, A) := g(v, w, A)$ otherwise. If we want to achieve an invariance of the energy under non-monotone grey-value transformation, the symmetry condition $g(v, w, A) = g(-v, w, A) = g(v, -w, A)$ has to be fulfilled.

Figure 1 shows results obtained for the registration of image morphologies. Here, we have considered an elastic regularization approach (cf. Section 4), to overcome the ill-posedness of the resulting matching problem.

3 Ill-posedness of the Problem

In general the image registration problem is not well-posed in the sense of Hadamard, i.e. for all admissible images one of the following properties does not hold

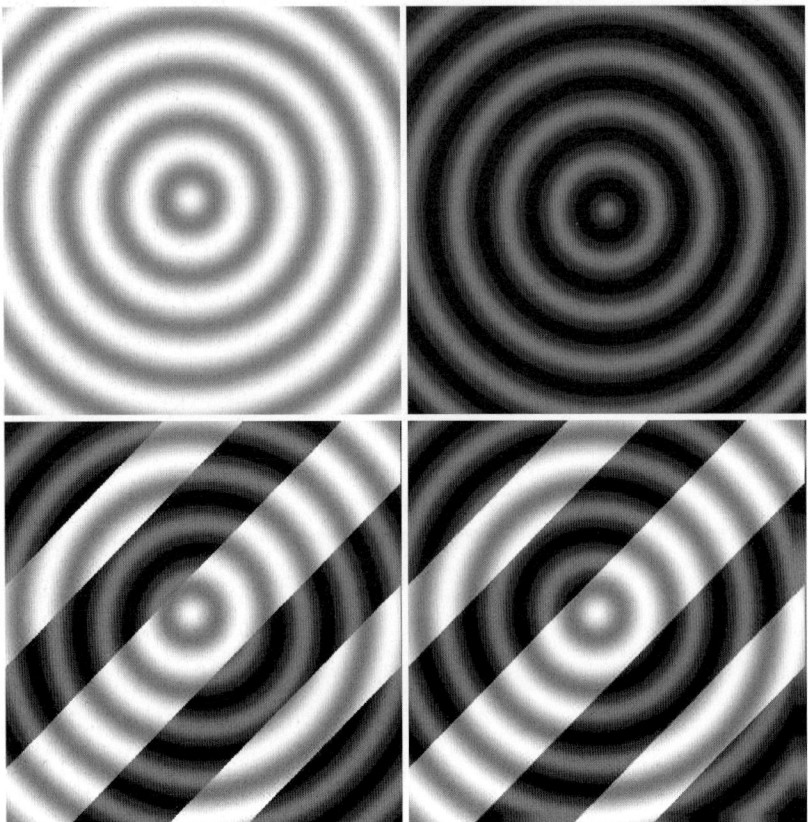

Fig. 1. An artificial test example for multi-modal morphological matching. The top row shows the given template resp. reference images which differ by a translation and a non-monotone contrast change. The bottom row depicts the initial misfit (left) and the final registration result by multi-scale minimization of the morphological registration energy.

(H1) a deformation exists,
(H2) the deformation is unique and
(H3) the deformation depends continuously on the images.

In practice the violation of the existence of a deformation does not play an important role. For instance, in the case of mono-modal matching almost all practical problems do not have an exact solution. To overcome this issue our aim is weakened by:

$$T \circ \phi \approx R.$$

The most often used strategy to solve the above "equation" is the definition of an energy, which leads for global minimizers (or maximizers) to an almost perfect matching result. Furthermore one designs these energies such that certain additional assumptions are fulfilled, as e.g. invariance w.r.t. rigid body motions and/or higher regularity [13].

The violation of the uniqueness of a deformation is a much more serious problem for the user as well as for the mathematician. In order to demonstrate this for the mono-modal matching problem, we consider the setting with the L^2-distance D^{LSQ}.

For a deformation ϕ and for $c \in \mathbb{R}$ the level sets

$$\mathcal{M}_c^T = \{x \in \Omega \mid T(x) = c\}$$

any displacement Λ which keeps $\mathcal{M}_c^T$ fixed for all c, does not change the energy, i.e.,

$$D[\phi] = D[\Lambda \circ \phi].$$

This especially holds true for a possible minimizer ϕ. Hence, a minimizer – if it exists – is non-unique and the set of minimizers is expected to be non-regular and not closed in a usual set of admissible displacements. Note that the above example holds for all energies which are based on the matching of level-sets.

The problem is turning even worse in case of multi-modal registration problems. Indeed, for any deformation ϕ which maps level sets onto level set ($T(x) = T(y) \Rightarrow T \circ \phi(x) = T \circ \phi(y)$) - not necessary corresponding ones - we then still have that $D[\phi] = D[\Lambda \circ \phi]$.

Since the image registration problem has obviously multiple solutions and the solution set is typically very large and irregular one has to decide which solution is of interest (for a given application) and which is not. From the mathematical point of view, the problem behaves just like a singular system. Generically, there is not enough information to determine a deformation uniquely. The problem is underdetermined. Additional information will be inserted most commonly requiring "smoothness" of a solution.

4 Regularization of the Problem

The aim of this section is to introduce different minimization approaches to the problem

$$D[\cdot] \longrightarrow \min. \tag{2}$$

Most common approaches to minimize nonlinear functionals are steepest decent and Newton type methods. Unfortunately, even when (H2) is fulfilled, the use of this methods leads to serious numerical problems, since a solution of the image registration problem does not depend continuously on the image-data.

Unfortunately, recalling our observation above irregular in particular discontinuous solutions with arbitrary large strain are possible. To rule out these unrequested solutions it is necessary to penalize them.

4.1 Energy Relaxation

One way of doing so consists in changing the energy functional and adding a so called regularization energy. Typical examples of such energies are

- a Dirichlet functional
$$S^{Dir}[\phi] = \int_\Omega |\nabla \phi|^2 \, dx, \tag{3}$$

which indeed leads to better smoothness properties of the results. Nagel and Enkelmann proposed an anisotropic quadratic form for the gradient of the deformation which regularizes edges of the image only in the tangential direction [11, 26]. Alvarez, Weickert and Sanchez [2] used these ideas for deriving a consistent model, centering deformation and anisotropy in the same image.
- functionals from elasticity, which relates to the assumption that the deformation is caused by some kind of elastic forces. The structure of those energies for $n = 3$ is as follows:
$$S^{elast}[\phi] = \int_\Omega W(D\phi, \mathrm{cof} D\phi, \det D\phi) \, dx. \tag{4}$$

In the above integrand we use the cofactor matrix $\mathrm{cof} D\phi$ of the derivative $D\phi$ and the corresponding determinant.
- higher order functionals. Here a well known example is used in [13]
$$S^{higher}[\phi] = \sum_{l=1}^d \int_\Omega |\Delta \phi_l|^2 \, dx, \tag{5}$$

Note that the addition of those energies leads to minimizers which no longer yield perfect matching results. In this sense we weakened our aim and try to find almost perfect matches ϕ with
$$T \circ \phi \approx R.$$

Let us collect what we have found so far. We want to solve the image matching problem by minimizing an energy whose ingredients are the similarity measure and a regularization energy:
$$E[\phi] = D[\phi] + \alpha S[\phi] \tag{6}$$

This approach is in the inverse problem community widely known as Tikhonov regularization.

4.2 Iterative Relaxation

Henn and Witsch [18] introduced the so called iterative Tikhonov regularization for minimizing $D[u]$. The solution of the minimization problem is denoted by u_α for α fixed. Now, we consider a solution curve u_α for decreasing α. One starts with $\alpha_0 \gg 0$ which is helpful for the solution method. Then minimal solutions of the

Tikhonov functional

$$u^{k+1} = \arg\min_u \{D[u] + \alpha_k S(u - u^{(k)})\}$$

with a monotone decreasing sequence $\alpha_k \to 0$ for $k \to \infty$ and initial guess $u^{(k)}$ are computed. Each subproblem, for regular chosen S and α_k sufficiently large, is well posed. The iteration is stopped whenever the functional D increases.

At the end of this section we want to consider a different related regularization method, based on gradient flow ideas. Gradient flows are well known tools in minimization of functionals. Classical examples are the heat flow as gradient flow for the Dirichlet integral or mean curvature evolution of surfaces as a gradient flow for the area-functional (see e.g. [22]).

Here, we want to describe a gradient flow approach to the minimization problem (2), i.e., we would like to determine a path within a suitable space of deformations, that tends towards the set of minima of D.

On account of the discussed ill-posedness of this problem, gradient flows have to integrate regularizations to avoid nonsmooth paths on the energy landscape.

At this point, we see a principal difference between "classical" gradient flow methods [27] for PDEs and our approach to ill-posed optimization problems. We do not interpret a given PDE as a gradient flow but we use metrics for modeling and regularization purposes.

The idea is to introduce a regularizing metric $g : \mathcal{X} \times \mathcal{X} \to \mathbb{R}$ measuring the derivative of D in a regular space $\mathcal{X}$. If we consider the duality in $\mathcal{X}'$ we have a representation $A : \mathcal{X} \to \mathcal{X}'$ of g :

$$g(u,v) = \langle Au, v \rangle.$$

Obviously, this mapping is bijective on account of the metric properties. If we measure the derivative w.r.t. g then the formal gradient flow with respect to the metric $g(\cdot,\cdot)$

$$\partial_t u(t) = -\mathrm{grad}_g D[u(t)]$$

reads as

$$g(\partial_t u, \varphi) = -\langle D'[u], \varphi \rangle,$$

for all $\varphi \in \mathcal{X}$. This can be re-formulated using the mapping A ($A\,\partial_t u = -D'[u]$) or equivalently:

$$\partial_t u = -A^{-1} D'[u].$$

The mapping A^{-1} transfers the derivative of D to the more regular space $\mathcal{X}$. For more details and relations to the above regularization methods we refer to [8].

5 Computational Approaches to Minimize the Matching Energy

In the previous section we have discussed the image registration problem. It turns out, that the problem is ill-posed and consequently traditional numerical methods must fail. The aim of this section is to present some basic computational approaches to solve the image registration problem, i.e., to minimize a similarity functional D, or to find roots of

$$f(u) := \operatorname{grad} D[u].$$

Furthermore, we define an energy norm $\|\cdot\|_E$ defined by

$$\|v\|_E = \sqrt{\langle v, v \rangle_E}$$

with inner product

$$\langle v, w \rangle_E = \langle Av, w \rangle_{L_2^d(\Omega)} \tag{7}$$

and a symmetric positive definite operator A. Let us hint at the fact, that this energy norm can be regarded as regularizing metric as discussed above.

5.1 Direct Time Dependent Methods

One of the most basic ideas for the solution of the minimization of the similarity measure D consists in applying a steepest descent method. Thus we look for a path in the energy landscape of the deformations heading always in the direction $-\operatorname{grad} D[u]$. This direction interpreted in the metric sense is given by $-A^{-1}f(u)$. Continuously we consider the evolution problem

$$u_t + A^{-1}f(u) = 0, \quad 0 \leq t \leq T, \quad u(0) = u_0.$$

The easiest time-discretization is the following one:

1) **Explicit Time Discretization**
Here, the next iterate is given by simply going one timestep τ in the direction of the steepest descent (gradient direction):

$$\frac{u_{k+1} - u_k}{\tau} + A^{-1} f(u_k) = 0.$$

This is equivalent to the scheme

$$u_{k+1} = u_k - \tau A^{-1} f(u_k).$$

An additional line-search leads to a more efficient and stable method:

$$\tau_k = \arg\min_{\tau \in \mathbb{R}} D\left[u_k - \tau A^{-1} f(u_k)\right]. \tag{8}$$

Algorithmically, this reads as in Algorithm 4. Higher stability of the steepest descent method may be obtained by an

Algorithm 4 Steepest descent with explicit time discretization

1: $k = 0$; $u^{(0)} = 0$;
2: **repeat**
3:     calculate $f_k = f(u_k(x))$;
4:     compute $d_k = A^{-1} f_k$ with A given by (7);
5:     compute τ_k by solving problem (8);
6:     set $u_{k+1} = u_k + \tau_k \cdot d_k$;
7:     set $k = k + 1$;
8: **until** $||f(u_k)||^2 \leq eps$

2) **Implicit Time Discretization**

In this case, the descent direction is taken at time τ instead of the "old" time 0. Principally we have to solve a nonlinear problem.

$$\frac{u_{k+1} - u_k}{\tau} + A^{-1} f(u_{k+1}) = 0$$

Formally, the determination of the next time-step is similar to the explicit case:

$$u_{k+1} = u_k - \tau A^{-1} f(u_{k+1}),\,.$$

Nevertheless, such a fully implicit discretization is rarely applied because it is not really practical.

5.2 Regularized Time Dependent Methods

In the above solution methods we introduced a regularization via regularizing the descent direction using the representation A of the energy E. Another possibility consists in adding a regularization energy and minimizing the resulting energy:

$$J_\alpha(u) = D[u] + \alpha ||u||_E^2 \to min!$$

In this case, a descent direction of $J_\alpha(u)$ is given by $\alpha A u + f(u)$. In the same way as above, a continuous model leading to at least local minimizers is:

$$u_t + \alpha A u + f(u) = 0, \quad 0 \leq t \leq T, \quad u(0) = u_0\,.$$

3.) **Explicit time discretization**. Conceptually, there is no difference compared to the above explicit time discretization. The search direction is now given by $\alpha A u_k + f(u_k)$:

$$\frac{u_{k+1} - u_k}{\tau} + \alpha A u_k + f(u_k) = 0$$

The update displacement computes as:

$$u_{k+1} = u_k - \tau \underbrace{(\alpha A u_k + f(u_k))}_{=J'_\alpha}\,.$$

Once again a line-search algorithm as in (8) should be used for efficiency reasons.

Algorithm 5 Steepest descent with semi-implicit time discretization

$k = 0; u^{(0)} = 0;$
repeat
    calculate $f_k = f(u^{(k)}(x))$
    compute $l^{(k)} = u_k - \tau f_k$
    solve $(I + \alpha \tau A) u_{k+1} = l^{(k)}$
    set $k = k + 1$
until $||f(u^{(k)}(x))||^2 \leq eps$

4) **Semi-implicit Discretization**. One frequently used technique consists in treating the linear term Au implicitly and the nonlinear derivative of the difference measure explicitly:

$$\frac{u_{k+1} - u_k}{\tau} + \alpha A u_{k+1} + f(u_k) = 0.$$

As corresponding system which is to solve we obtain:

$$(I + \alpha \tau A) u_{k+1} = u_k - \tau f(u_k)$$

The displacement update is given by

$$u_{k+1} = u_k - \tau (I + \alpha \tau A)^{-1} (\alpha A u_k + f(u_k)).$$

Thus, $(I + \alpha \tau A)^{-1}(\alpha A u_k + f(u_k))$ is a descend direction of J_α (cf. Algorithm 5) As usual for non-explicit methods, a line-search algorithm is at least difficult to implement.

5) **Implicit Discretization**
The fully implicit highly nonlinear problem

$$\frac{u_{k+1} - u_k}{\tau} + \alpha A u_{k+1} + f(u_{k+1}) = 0$$

arising from a regularization of the energy is not used in practice.

5.3 Gradient Descent Methods

We start the discussion of minimization methods by considering the unconstraint minimization problem

$$\min_u D.$$

Mathematically, d_k is a descend direction from u_k if

$$\left\langle grad(D[u_k]), d_k \right\rangle < 0$$

and it is guaranteed that for sufficient small $\tau > 0$

$$D[u_k + \tau d_k] < D[u_k].$$

If d_k is a descend direction and $\tau > 0$ sufficient small, then

$$u^{k+1} = u_k + \tau d_k.$$

reduces the value of the matching energy D. This motivates the following iterative method for the image registration problem

$$u^{k+1} = u_k + \tau_k d_k$$

with a parameter τ_k chosen by a line-search method. Since the image registration problem is ill-conditioned, methods based on these descend directions do not even converge locally. Hence, to ensure robustness and fast local convergence it is necessary to incorporate additional information.

6) **Steepest Descent Method in terms of an Energy**

The direction of most rapid descend of D at u_k is the solution of

$$\min_d \langle grad(D[u_k]), d_k \rangle,$$

and is called the steepest descent direction

$$d_k = -grad(D[u_k]) = -f_k.$$

Consider the quadratic approximation of $D[u_k + d_k]$

$$Q_k[d_k] = D[u_k] + \langle grad(D[u_k]), d_k \rangle$$
$$+ \frac{1}{2} \langle H_D(u_k) d_k, d_k \rangle$$

with the Hessian $H_D(u_k)$ of D at u_k. Since the Hessian is in general for the image registration problem not positive definite, the minimization of Q_k has not a unique minimizer. Therefore the Hessian is replaced by a well known positive definite operator A and we get the following perturbed steepest descent direction

$$d_k = -grad_A(D) = -A^{-1} f_k. \qquad (9)$$

The next iterate is given by

$$u^{k+1} = u_k - \tau A^{-1} f_k, \quad k = 0, 1, \cdots$$

with

$$\tau_k = \arg\min_{\tau \in \mathbb{R}} D\left[u_k - \tau A^{-1} f_k\right]. \qquad (10)$$

We get the following algorithm.

Algorithm 6 Perturbed steepest descent method for D

$k = 0;\ u^{(0)} = 0;$
repeat
    calculate $f_k = f(u_k(x))$
    compute d_k from *(9)*
    set $s_k = d_k/\|d_k\|_\infty$
    compute τ_k by solving problem *(10)*
    set $u^{k+1} = u_k + \tau_k \cdot s_k$
    set $k = k + 1$
until $\|f(u_k(x))\|^2 \leq eps$

7) **Steepest Descent Method for J_α**
Consider the regularized functional

$$J_\alpha[u] = D[u] + \alpha \left\langle Au, u \right\rangle_{L_2^d(\Omega)}$$

the steepest descent direction of J_α at u_k is given by

$$d_k = -grad_{J_\alpha}(D[u_k]) = -(\alpha A u_k + f_k). \tag{11}$$

For a given initial guess $u^{(0)}$ we get the following iteration

$$u^{k+1} = u_k - \tau_k(\alpha A u_k + f_k), \quad k = 0, 1, \cdots$$

where the parameter τ_k is the solution of the following line-search problem

$$\tau_k = \arg\min_{\tau \in \mathbb{R}} J_\alpha\left[u_k - \tau(\alpha A u_k + f_k)\right]. \tag{12}$$

8) **Steepest Descent Method for J_α in terms of an Energy**
Consider the regularized functional

$$J_\alpha[u] = D[u] + \alpha \left\langle Au, u \right\rangle_{L_2^d(\Omega)}$$

Algorithm 7 Steepest descent method for the regularized functional $J_\alpha[u]$

$k = 0;\ u^{(0)} = 0;$
repeat
    calculate $f_k = f(u_k(x))$
    compute d_k from *(11)*
    compute τ_k by solving problem *(12)*
    set $u^{k+1} = u_k - \tau_k(\alpha A u_k + f_k)$
    set $k = k + 1$
until $\|\alpha A u_k + f_k\|^2 \leq eps$

Algorithm 8 Perturbed steepest descent method for $J_\alpha[u]$

$k = 0$; $u^{(0)} = 0$;
repeat
    calculate $f_k = f(u_k(x))$
    compute d_k from *(13)*
    compute τ_k by solving problem *(14)*
    set $u^{k+1} = u_k - \tau_k(\alpha u_k + A^{-1} f_k)$
    set $k = k + 1$
until $\|\alpha A u_k + f_k\|^2 \leq eps$

a quadratic approximation of $J_\alpha[u_k + d_k]$ is given by

$$Q_k[d_k] = J_\alpha[u_k] + \left\langle grad(J_\alpha[u_k]), d_k \right\rangle$$

$$+ \frac{1}{2} \left\langle H_J[u_k] d_k, d_k \right\rangle$$

with the Hessian $H_J(u_k) = H_D(u_k) + \alpha A$ of J at u_k. Since $H_D(u_k)$ is ill-conditioned, we replace $H_J(u_k)$ by A and get the following quadratic approximation

$$Q_k[d_k] = J[u_k] + \left\langle grad(J[u_k]), d_k \right\rangle$$

$$+ \frac{1}{2} \left\langle A(u_k) d_k, d_k \right\rangle$$

with unique minimizer

$$d_k = -A^{-1}(\alpha A u_k + f_k) = -\alpha u_k - A^{-1} f_k \qquad (13)$$

for a given initial guess $u^{(0)}$ we get the following iteration

$$\begin{aligned} u^{k+1} &= u_k - \tau(\alpha u_k + A^{-1} f_k) \\ &= (1 - \alpha\tau) u_k - \tau A^{-1} f_k, \quad k = 0, 1, \cdots \end{aligned}$$

with τ_k solution of

$$\tau_k = \arg\min_{\tau \in \mathbb{R}} J_\alpha \left[u_k - \tau(\alpha u_k + A^{-1} f_k) \right]. \qquad (14)$$

A different approach uses the regularized functional. The reason is that higher values of α can be used without increasing the regularization. This yields derivatives with better condition. The first approach is given by:

10) Consider the regularized functional

$$J_\alpha^k[u] = D[u] + \alpha \left\langle A(u - u_k), u - u_k \right\rangle_{L_2^d(\Omega)}$$

with steepest descent direction

$$\mathrm{grad}_{J_\alpha^k}(D[u]) = f(u) + \alpha A(u - u_k)$$

of $J_\alpha[u]$. The evaluation at u_k leads to

$$d_k = -\mathrm{grad}\left(J_\alpha^k[u_k]\right) = -f_k.$$

This approach lead to the steepest descend iteration for D

$$u^{k+1} = u_k - \tau f_k$$

with a line-search

$$\tau_k = \arg\min_{\tau \in \mathbb{R}} J_\alpha\left[(u_k - \tau f_k)\right].$$

over the regularized functional J_α.
11) Consider the regularized functional

$$J_\alpha^k[u] = D[u] + \alpha \left\langle A(u - u_k), u - u_k \right\rangle_{L_2^d(\Omega)}$$

by replacing the Hessian of J_α^k by A we get the unique descend direction at u_k

$$d_k = -A^{-1} f_k$$

for a given initial guess $u^{(0)}$ we get the following iteration

$$u^{k+1} = u_k - \tau A^{-1} f_k, \quad k = 0, 1, \cdots$$

with

$$\tau_k = \arg\min_{\tau \in \mathbb{R}} J_\alpha^k\left[u_k - \tau A^{-1} f_k\right].$$

5.4 Higher Order Methods

In the case that the similarity functional is given by a least-squares functional, such as

$$D^{LSQ}[u(x)] = \frac{1}{2} \int_\Omega \left(T(x + u(x)) - R(x)\right)^2 dx$$

higher order minimization methods can be considered.

Newton-type methods An affine model of $d(u) = T(x - u(x)) - R(x)$ around a vector u_k is given by

$$d(u) - d(u_k) \approx J_d(u_k) \underbrace{(u - u_k)}_{=d_k}, \tag{15}$$

where J_d is the Jacobian of d given by

$$J_d(u) = \left(\frac{\partial d(u)}{\partial u_1}, \ldots, \frac{\partial d(u)}{\partial u_d}\right).$$

The Jacobian matrix and the Hessian of D^{LSQ} at u_k are given by

$$g(u_k) = J_d^t(u_k)d(u_k)$$

and

$$H(u_k) = J_d^t(u_k)J_d(u_k) + S(u_k).$$

Here,

$$S(u) = \int_\Omega d(u)d''(u)dx = \int_\Omega d(u)\nabla^2 T(x - u(x))dx$$

constitutes the nonlinear part of $H(u)$.

Newton-type methods applied on the image registration problem are iterative methods which can be written as:

$$u^{k+1} = u_k + d_k,$$

at each step, where $u^{(0)}$ is an initial given vector and d_k is the solution of the normal equation:

$$d_k = -A_k^{-1}g(u_k) = -A_k^{-1}J_d^t(u_k)d(u_k).$$

In the case $A_k = I$ this is just the steepest descend method. Higher order methods are given by:

- $A_k = H(u_k)$ Newton's method
- $A_k = J_d^t(u_k) \cdot J_d(u_k)$ Gauss-Newton method.

For the most real applications these methods are not suitable to solve the registration problem. The matrix A_k has a large condition number $cond_2(A_k)$ so that these methods do not even converge locally and due to noise sensitivity of the ill-posed problem, regularization techniques have to be applied in order to compute meaningful solutions. The modified Newton step

$$d_k = -(J_d^t(u_k) \cdot J_d(u_k) + \alpha_k A)^{-1} J_d^t(u_k)d(u_k) \tag{16}$$

becomes well posed for some $\alpha_k > 0$ with unknown size. A trust-region approach to determine the parameter α_k in each iteration step is presented in [17].

Nonlinear Approaches Here the idea is to minimize the nonlinear regularized functional

$$J_\alpha[u] = D[u] + \alpha ||u||_E^2$$

by a nonlinear iterative method. Amit [3] uses Fourier and Wavelet techniques. In [18] an approach is presented, where the multigrid-idea and the minimization of the nonlinear functional is combined by a modified multigrid full approximation scheme.

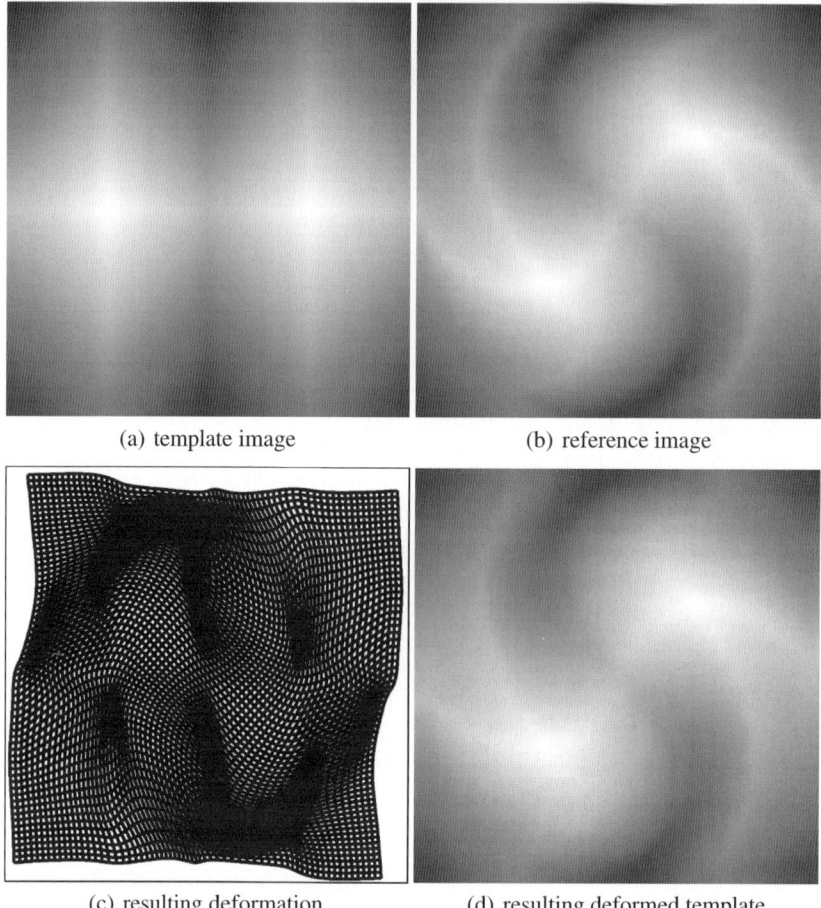

Fig. 2. Example for a multiscale uni-modal image registration problem with large deformation: The reference (b) is an artificial rotational distortion of the template (a). The computation of the result involved gradient descents on the complete hierarchy of grids.

5.5 Multi-scale Approaches

At the end of this section we want to hint at a well-established global minimizing approaches for image matching problems, based on a multi-scale of matching problems.

For typical image intensity functions T, R, as discussed above the energy $D[\cdot]$ is non-convex and we expect an energy landscape with many local minima. Especially for gradient flow methods this implies that descent paths mostly tend to asymptotic states which only locally minimize the energy. Following Alvarez et al. [1] we consider a continuous annealing method based on a whole scale of image pairs T_ϵ, R_ϵ, where $\epsilon \geq 0$ is the scale parameter. Here we consider scale spaces of images generated by a scale space operator $S(\cdot)$ which maps an initial image I onto some coarser image, i.e.,

$$I_\epsilon = S(\epsilon) I .$$

The scale parameter ϵ allows to select fine grain representations corresponding to small values of ϵ and coarse grain representations with most of the image details skipped for larger values of ϵ. For the choice of S we refer to [7, section 4, 6]. For given $\epsilon \geq 0$ we then consider the difference measure

$$D_\epsilon[u] = \frac{1}{2} \int_\Omega |T_\epsilon \circ (\mathbb{1} + u) - R_\epsilon|^2 .$$

We are left to choose the initial mapping $\phi_0 = \mathbb{1} + u_{0,\epsilon}$ for the evolution on scale ϵ. Here we expect the minimizer or a sufficiently good approximation of the same problem on a coarse scale to be a suitable starting point to approach the global minimum on the finer scale. Thus, in an iteration, starting from a coarse scale with large value of ϵ, one successively refines the small and reduces ϵ correspondingly. Details of the implementation are given in [7, section 4, 6]. An example with a large non-linear deformation, where computations took place from coarse to fine scales resolved on suitably resolved grids is given in Figure 2, where the template and reference images differ by a rotational twist by up to $\frac{\pi}{4}$.

References

1. L. Alvarez, J. Weickert J. and Sánchez: A scale–space approach to nonlocal optical flow calculations, M. Nielsen, P. Johansen, O. F. Olsen and J. Weickert (Eds), Scale-Space Theories in Computer Vision. Second International Conference, Scale-Space '99, Corfu, Greece, September 1999, Lecture Notes in Computer Science, **1682**, pp 235-246, Springer, (1999)
2. L. Alvarez, J. Weickert and J. Sánchez: Reliable estimation of dense optical flow fields with large displacements, International Journal of Computer Vision, **39**, pp 41-56, (2000)
3. Y. Amit: A nonlinear variational problem for image matching, SIAM J. Sci. Comput., **15**, pp 207-224, (1994)
4. K. Cattermole: Statistische Analyse und Struktur von Information, VCH, (1988)
5. G. E. Christensen, S. C. Joshi and M. I. Miller: Volumetric transformations of brain anatomy, IEEE Trans. Medical Imaging, **16/6**, pp 864-877, (1997)
6. G. E. Christensen, R. D. Rabbitt and M. I. Miller: Deformable templates using large deformation kinematics, IEEE Trans. Medical Imaging, **5/10**, pp 1435-1447, (1996)
7. U. Clarenz, M. Droske and M. Rumpf: Towards fast non-rigid registration, Preprint, (2002)
8. U. Clarenz, S. Henn, M. Rumpf and K. Witsch: Relations between optimization and gradient flow methods with applications to image registration, Proceedings of the 18th GAMM Seminar Leipzig on Multigrid and Related Methods for Optimisation Problems, pp 11–30, (2002)
9. E. D'Agostino, J. Modersitzki, F. Maes, D. Vandermeulen, B. Fischer and P. Suetens: Free-form registration using mutual information and curvature regularization, Preprint A-03-05, Institute of Mathematics, Medical University of Lübeck, (2003)

10. C. A. Davatzikos, R. N. Bryan and J. L. Prince: Image registration based on boundary mapping, IEEE Trans. Medical Imaging, **15/1**, pp 112-115, (1996)
11. R. Deriche, P. Kornobst and G. Aubert: Optical–flow estimation while preserving its discontinuities: A variational approach, Proc. Second Asian Conf. Computer Vision (ACCV '95, Singapore, December 5–8, 1995), **2**, pp 290-295, (1995)
12. M. Droske, and M. Rumpf: A variational approach to non-rigid morphological registration, SIAM Appl. Math., **64/2**, pp 668-687, (2004)
13. B. Fischer J. and Modersitzki: Curvature based image registration, Journal of Mathematic Imaging and Vision, **18/1**, pp 81-85, (2003)
14. G. Hermosillo, C. Chefd'hotel and O. Faugeras: Variational methods for multi-modal image matching, Int. J. Comput. Vision, **50/3**, pp 329-343, (2002)
15. U. Grenander and M. I. Miller: Computational anatomy: An emerging discipline, Quarterly Appl. Math., LVI, **4**, pp 617-694, (1998)
16. Hanke, M. and Groetsch, C. W.: Nonstationary iterated tikhonov regularization, J. Optim. Theory and Applications, **98**, pp 37-53, (1998)
17. S. Henn: A Levenberg-Marquardt Scheme for nonlinear image registration, BIT Numerical Mathematics, **43/4**, pp 743-759, (2003)
18. S. Henn and K. Witsch: Iterative multigrid regularization techniques for image matching, SIAM J. Sci. Comput. (SISC), **23/4**, pp 1077-1093, (2001)
19. S. Henn and K. Witsch: Multi-modal image registration using a variational approach, SIAM J. Sci. Comput. (SISC), **25/4**, pp 1429-1447, (2004)
20. G. Hermosillo: Variational methods for multi-modal image matching, Phd thesis, Université de Nice, France, (2002)
21. G. Hermosillo, C. Chef d'Hotel and O. Faugeras: Variational methods for multi-modal image matching, International Journal of Computer Vision, **50/3**, pp 329-343, (December 2002)
22. G. Huisken: The volume preserving mean curvature flow, J. Reine Angew. Math., **382**, pp 35-48, (1987)
23. S. C. Joshi and M. I. Miller: Landmark matching via large deformation diffeomorphisms, IEEE Trans. Medical Imaging, **9/8**, pp 1357-1370, (2000)
24. F. Maes, A. Collignon, D. Vandermeulen, G. Marchal and P. Suetens: Multi-modality image registration maximization of mutual information, Proceedings of the 1996 Workshop on Mathematical Methods in Biomedical Image Analysis (MMBIA '96), pp 14. IEEE Computer Society, (1996)
25. F. Maes, A. Collignon, D. Vandermeulen, G. Marchal and P. Suetens: Multi–modal volume registration by maximization of mutual information, IEEE Trans. Medical Imaging, **16/7**, pp 187-198, (1997)
26. H. H. Nagel and W. Enkelmann: An investigation of smoothness constraints for the estimation of displacement vector fields from image sequences, IEEE Trans. Pattern Anal. Mach. Intell., **8**, pp 565-593, (1986)
27. F. Otto: The geometry of dissipative evolution equation: the porous medium equation, Comm. Partial Differential Equations, **26/1-2**, pp 101-174, (2001)
28. E. Radmoser, O. Scherzer and J. Weickert: Scale–space properties of regularization methods, M. Nielsen, P. Johansen, O. F. Olsen and J. Weickert (Eds), Scale-Space Theories in Computer Vision. Second International Conference, Scale-Space '99, Corfu, Greece, September 1999, Lecture Notes in Computer Science; Springer, **1682**, pp 211-220, (1999)
29. K. Rohr, H.S. Stiehl, R. Sprengel, W. Beil, T. M. Buzug, J. Weese and M. H. Kuhn: Point-based elastic registration of medical image data using approximating thin-plate splines, Lecture Notes in Computer Science, **1131**, pp 297-306, (1996)

30. G. Sapiro: Geometric Partial Differential Equations and Image Processing, Cambridge University Press, (2001)
31. O. Scherzer and J. Weickert: Relations between regularization and diffusion filtering, (1998)
32. J. P. Thirion: Image matching as a diffusion process: An analogy with maxwell's demon, Medical Imag. Analysis, **2**, pp 243-260, (1998)
33. P. Thompson and A. Toga: Anatomically driven strategies for high-dimensional brain image registration and pathology, Brain Warping, Academic Press, pp 311-336, (1998)
34. P. A. Viola: Alignment by maximization of mutual information, Technical Report AITR-1548, (1995)
35. J. Weickert: Anisotropic diffusion in image processing, Teubner, (1998)
36. W. Wells, P. Viola, H. Atsumi, S. Nakajima and R. Kikinis: Multi-modal volume registration by maximization of mutual information, Medical Image Analysis, **1**, pp 35-51, (1996)

A Survey on Variational Optic Flow Methods for Small Displacements

Joachim Weickert[1], Andrés Bruhn[1], Thomas Brox[1], and Nils Papenberg[2]

[1] Mathematical Image Analysis Group, Faculty of Mathematics and Computer Science, Saarland University, Building 27, 66041 Saarbrücken, Germany {weickert, bruhn, brox}@mia.uni-saarland.de
[2] Institute of Mathematics, University of Lübeck, Wallstraße 40, 23560 Lübeck, Germany, papenber@math.uni-luebeck.de

Summary Optic flow describes the displacement field in an image sequence. Its reliable computation constitutes one of the main challenges in computer vision, and variational methods belong to the most successful techniques for achieving this goal. Variational methods recover the optic flow field as a minimiser of a suitable energy functional that involves data and smoothness terms. In this paper we present a survey on different model assumptions for each of these terms and illustrate their impact by experiments. We restrict ourselves to rotationally invariant convex functionals with a linearised data term. Such models are appropriate for small displacements. Regarding the data term, constancy assumptions on the brightness, the gradient, the Hessian, the gradient magnitude, the Laplacian, and the Hessian determinant are investigated. Local integration and nonquadratic penalisation are considered in order to improve robustness under noise. With respect to the smoothness term, we review a recent taxonomy that links regularisers to diffusion processes. It allows to distinguish five types of regularisation strategies: homogeneous, isotropic image-driven, anisotropic image-driven, isotropic flow-driven, and anisotropic flow-driven. All these regularisations can be performed either in the spatial or the spatiotemporal domain. After discussing well-posedness results for convex optic flow functionals, we sketch some numerical ideas in order to achieve real-time performance on a standard PC by means of multigrid methods, and we survey a simple and intuitive confidence measure.

1 Introduction

Finding the displacement field between subsequent frames of an image sequence has become a classical computer vision problem. This displacement field is called *optic flow*. Solving the optic flow problem does not only have an impact in fields like video coding or robot navigation, it is also a prototype for the entire class of correspondence problems, where one seeks a sufficiently smooth mapping that maps the features in one image to the structures in another one. Other applications where such problems appear include the fields of stereo reconstruction and medical image registration.

Already in 1981, Horn and Schunck introduced the first variational method for computing the optic flow field in an image sequence [44]. This method is based on two assumptions that are characteristic for many variational optic flow methods: a brightness constancy assumption and a smoothness assumption. These assumptions enter a continuous energy functional whose minimiser yields the desired optic flow field.

Performance evaluations such as [9, 35] showed that variational methods belong to the best performing techniques for computing the optic flow field. It is thus not surprising that a lot of research has been carried out in order to improve these techniques even further: These amendments include refined model assumptions with discontinuity-preserving constraints [2, 28, 42, 62, 65, 73, 91] or spatiotemporal regularisation [11, 61, 92], improved data terms with modified constraints [3, 26, 62, 74] or nonquadratic penalisation [11, 43, 56, 26], and efficient multigrid algorithms [15, 22, 39, 38, 78, 95] for minimising these energy functionals.

The goal of the present chapter is to analyse the data term and the smoothness term in detail and to survey some of our recent results on variational optic flow computation. For the sake of simplicity we focus on small displacements, where Taylor linearisations of the data term are valid approximations. This restriction allows to consider convex functionals where many theoretical and practical aspects become significantly easier and more transparent.

Our chapter is organised as follows: In Section 2 we sketch the general structure of these techniques. While Section 3 analyses the data term in more detail, a discussion of the different possibilities for smoothness constraints is given in Section 4. Suitable combinations of data and smoothness tersm are investigated in Section 5, well-posedness results are presented in Section 6, and algorithmic aspects are sketched in Section 7. A simple but general confidence measure for energy-based optic flow methods in discussed in Section 8. Our chapter is concluded with a summary in Section 9. A significantly shorter early version of the present chapter has been presented at a workshop [90].

2 General Structure

Let $f(x_1, x_2, x_3)$ denote some scalar-valued image sequence, where (x_1, x_2) is the location and x_3 denotes time. Often f is obtained by preprocessing some initial image sequence f_0 by convolving it with a Gaussian K_σ of standard deviation σ:

$$f = K_\sigma * f_0. \tag{1}$$

Let us assume that $D^k f$ describes the set of all partial (spatial and temporal) derivatives of f of order k, and that the optic flow field $u(x_1, x_2, x_3) = (u_1(x_1, x_2, x_3), u_2(x_1, x_2, x_3), 1)^\top$ gives the displacement rate between subsequent frames with temporal frame distance 1. In the present paper we consider variational methods that are based on the minimisation of the continuous energy functional

$$E(u) = \int_\Omega (\underbrace{M(D^k f, u)}_{\text{data term}} + \alpha \underbrace{S(\nabla f, \nabla u)}_{\text{regulariser}}) \, dx \qquad (2)$$

where the integration domain Ω is either a spatial or a spatiotemporal domain. In the spatial case we have $x := (x_1, x_2)^\top$ and $\nabla := \nabla_2 := (\partial_{x_1}, \partial_{x_2})^\top$, and in the spatiotemporal case we use the notations $x := (x_1, x_2, x_3)^\top$ and $\nabla := \nabla_3 := (\partial_{x_1}, \partial_{x_2}, \partial_{x_3})^\top$. The optic flow field $u(x_1, x_2, x_3)$ is obtained as a function that minimises $E(u)$. The energy functional $E(u)$ penalises all deviations from model assumptions. Typically is consists of a *data term* $M(D^k f, u)$ which expresses e.g. a brightness constancy assumption, and a *regulariser* $S(\nabla f, \nabla u)$ with $\nabla u := (\nabla u_1, \nabla u_2)^\top$ that penalises deviations from (piecewise) smoothness. The weight $\alpha > 0$ serves as *regularisation parameter:* Larger values correspond to more simplified flow fields.

The simplest and oldest representative of the class (2) is given by the method of Horn and Schunck [44]. It is based on the minimisation of the spatial functional

$$E(u) = \int_\Omega \left((u^\top \nabla_3 f)^2 + \alpha \sum_{i=1}^{2} |\nabla u_i|^2 \right) dx. \qquad (3)$$

As will be detailed in the forthcoming sections, the Horn–Schunck functional combines a data term that describes the brighness constancy of moving patterns with a smoothness term which involves homogeneous (Tikhonov [79]) regularisation.

It should be noted that continuous energy functionals of type (2) may be formulated in a rotationally invariant way: Apart from very few exceptions such as [6, 28, 52], almost all continuous optic flow functionals that have been proposed are rotationally invariant. Results from numerical analysis then show that consistent discretisations approximate this invariance under rotations arbitrarily well if the sampling is sufficiently fine. Moreover, if the energy functional is convex, a unique minimiser exists that can be found in a relatively simple way by globally convergent algorithms. Variational optic flow methods are *global* methods: If there is not sufficient local information, the data term $M(D^k f, u)$ is so small that it is dominated by the smoothness term $\alpha S(\nabla f, \nabla u)$ which fills in information from more reliable surrounding locations. Thus, in contrast to local methods, the *filling-in effect* of global variational approaches always yields dense flow fields and no subsequent interpolation steps are necessary: Everything is automatically accomplished within a single variational framework.

3 Data Terms

In the design of data terms for optic flow methods prior knowledge plays an important role. This knowledge may include information on the imaging device (e.g. the quality of the images with respect to noise), on the conditions during the acquisition of the video material (e.g. the occurrence of frequent illumination changes) as well as information on the expected type of motion (e.g. mainly translational motion of cars in traffic sequences). For a specific problem, this information may allow to select a data term that is especially appropriate and thus improves the quality of the estimation significantly. For this reason, the following section gives an overview on data terms that are frequently used in literature. Moreover, a detailed discussion on their advantages and shortcomings should guide the reader to select an appropriate data term for a specific problem.

3.1 Constancy Assumptions

In order to analyse motion within subsequent frames of an image sequence, temporal constancy has to be imposed on certain image features. The most frequently used feature in this context is the image brightness. Many differential methods are based on the assumption that this brightness is constant, i.e. that the grey value of objects does not change over time. If we denote the motion of some image structure by $(x_1(x_3), x_2(x_3))^\top$ this assumptions can be formulated as

$$\frac{df(x_1(x_3), x_2(x_3), x_3)}{dx_3} = 0. \qquad (4)$$

By applying the chain rule and defining $f_{x_i} := \partial_{x_i} f$ the following *optic flow constraint (OFC)* is obtained:

$$f_{x_1} u_1 + f_{x_2} u_2 + f_{x_3} = 0. \qquad (5)$$

Note that the optic flow field satisfies $(u_1, u_2, 1)^\top = (\partial_{x_3} x_1, \partial_{x_3} x_2, 1)^\top$.
It also is instructive to derive this constraint in a second way: Assuming a frame distance of 1, the brightness constancy constraint between two subsequent frames at time x_3 and $x_3 + 1$ can be expressed as

$$0 = f(x_1+u_1, x_2+u_2, x_3+1) - f(x_1, x_2, x_3) \qquad (6)$$

such that (5) follows from a Taylor linearisation in the point $(x_1, x_2, x_3)^\top$. However, this Taylor linearisation is only a reasonable approximation if the flow field varies sufficiently smooth and the displacement rates are small, i.e. in the order of one pixel or below. In the following we assume that this is the case, because it would be much more burdensome to deal with the unlinearised constraint (6) than its linearised counterpart (5).

In order to use equation (5) within the energy functional (2), we penalise all deviations from zero by considering the quadratic data term [44]

$$M_1(D^1 f, u) := (u^\top \nabla_3 f)^2. \qquad (7)$$

As long as the image data does not violate the brightness constancy assumption, the use of M_1 can give good results. In particular with regard to image data with non-constant brightness, however, constancy assumptions should be based on image features that are less sensitive to illumination changes. A simple and efficient strategy in this context is the consideration of derivatives. Instead of imposing constancy to the image brightness f along the path $(x_1(x_3), x_2(x_3))^\top$, one may e.g. assume that the spatial brightness gradient $(f_{x_1}, f_{x_2})^\top$ does not change along the same path [83]:

$$\frac{df_{x_1}(x_1(x_3), x_2(x_3), x_3)}{dx_3} = 0, \tag{8}$$

$$\frac{df_{x_2}(x_1(x_3), x_2(x_3), x_3)}{dx_3} = 0. \tag{9}$$

This gives the two equations

$$u^\top \nabla_3 f_{x_1} = 0, \tag{10}$$
$$u^\top \nabla_3 f_{x_2} = 0. \tag{11}$$

Squaring and adding them produces the data term

$$M_2(D^2 f, u) := \sum_{i=1}^{2} (u^\top \nabla_3 f_{x_i})^2. \tag{12}$$

In a straightforward way, constancy assumptions can also be imposed on higher-order derivatives, e.g. on the (spatial) Hessian $\mathcal{H}_2 f$. Squaring and adding the corresponding equations we obtain the following data term:

$$M_3(D^3 f, u) := \sum_{i=1}^{2} \sum_{j=1}^{2} (u^\top \nabla_3 f_{x_i x_j})^2. \tag{13}$$

With M_2 and M_3 we have proposed data terms that are designed for sequences with illumination changes. However, one should note that their performance depends significantly on the occurring type of motion. This has the following reason: In contrast to the image brightness both gradient and Hessian contain directional information. As a consequence, any constancy assumption on these expressions implies a constancy assumption on their orientation. On one hand, this property may be useful if it comes to the estimation of translational, divergent or slow rotational motion. In this case the orientation of the features does hardly change and the combination of two or three constraints in one data term may improve the results. On the other hand, poor results have to be expected if fast rotations are dominating and the implied orientation constancy does not hold.

A way to overcome this limitation is to create motion invariant image features from these "oriented" derivatives. Instead of imposing constancy on the (spatial) brightness gradient and therewith on its orientation, one may e.g. assume that only its magnitude is constant over time. Then, the following data term is obtained:

$$M_4(D^2 f, u) := (u^\top \nabla_3 |\nabla f|)^2. \tag{14}$$

This idea can also be extended to higher-order derivatives. As an example, let us consider the (spatial) Hessian $\mathcal{H}_2 f$. In this case, one may either think of imposing constancy on the (spatial) Laplacian $\Delta_2 f$ or on the determinant of the (spatial) Hessian $\mathcal{H}_2 f$. While the data term associated to the Laplacian is given by

$$M_5(D^3 f, u) := (u^\top \nabla_3 (\Delta_2 f))^2, \tag{15}$$

the data term based on the constancy of the determinant of the Hessian reads

$$M_6(D^3 f, u) := (u^\top \nabla_3 \det(\mathcal{H}_2 f))^2. \tag{16}$$

This example shows that in general multiple of such scalar valued expressions can be derived from the set of derivatives of a single order. However, there is no general rule which expression gives the best performance. An overview of all data terms presented so far is given in Table 1. It may also be useful to combine multiple of these terms by means of a linear combination. Moreover, one should note that M_2–M_6 can be more sensitive to noise than M_1, since they involve higher orders of derivatives of the image sequence.

In Figure 1 we illustrate the impact of different constancy assumptions on the computed flow field. To this end we use the data terms M_1–M_6 within a spatial energy functional based on homogeneous regularisation of Horn–Schunck type, i.e. we minimise

$$E(u) = \int_\Omega \left(M_j + \alpha \sum_{i=1}^{2} |\nabla u_i|^2 \right) dx. \tag{17}$$

Table 1. Comparison of the data terms M_1–M_6.

	data term	constancy assumption	illum. changes	motion type
M_1	$(u^\top \nabla_3 f)^2$	brightness	no	any
M_2	$\sum_{i=1}^{2} (u^\top \nabla_3 f_{x_i})^2$	gradient	yes	translational divergent slow rotational
M_3	$\sum_{i=1}^{2}\sum_{j=1}^{2} (u^\top \nabla_3 f_{x_i x_j})^2$	Hessian	yes	translational divergent slow rotational
M_4	$(u^\top \nabla_3 |\nabla f|)^2$	gradient magnitude	yes	any
M_5	$(u^\top \nabla_3 (\Delta_2 f))^2$	Laplacian	yes	any
M_6	$(u^\top \nabla_3 \det(\mathcal{H}_2 f))^2$	Hessian determinant	yes	any

A Survey on Variational Optic Flow Methods for Small Displacements

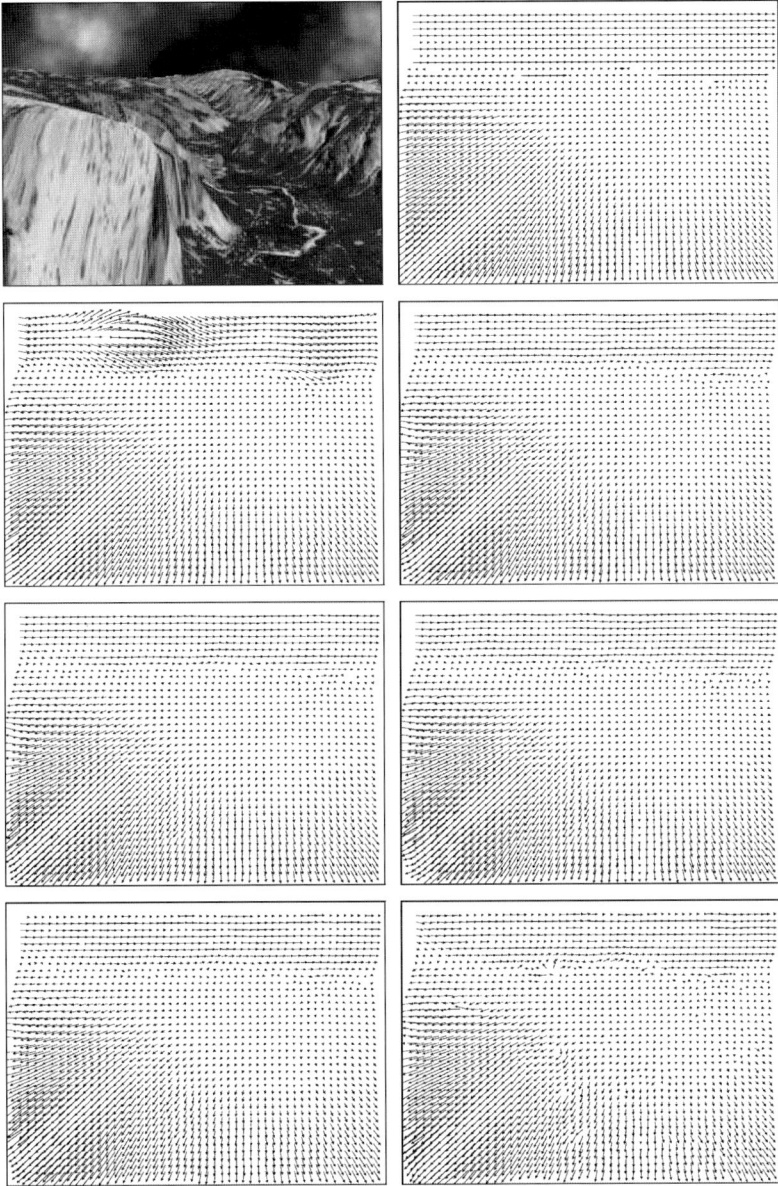

Fig. 1. *From left to right, and from top to bottom:* (a) Frame 8 of the Yosemite sequence *with clouds* of size 316×256. (b) Ground truth. (c) Computed flow field for a spatial approach with data term M_1 (brightness constancy) and homogeneous regularisation as smoothness term. (d) Data term M_2 (gradient constancy). (e) Data term M_3 (constancy of Hessian). (f) Data term M_4 (gradient magnitude constancy). (g) Data term M_5 (constancy of Laplacian). (h) Data term M_6 (constancy of Hessian determinant).

Table 2. Impact of the constancy assumption on the quality of the optic flow field. We used a spatial energy functional with homogeneous regularisation, and computed the average angular error (AAE) for the Yosemite sequence with clouds. The parameters σ and α have been optimised.

constancy assumption	data term	σ	α	AAE
brightness	M_1	1.30	500	7.17°
gradient	M_2	2.10	20	5.91°
Hessian	M_3	2.70	1.8	6.46°
gradient magnitude	M_4	1.90	14	6.37°
Laplacian	M_5	2.50	3.0	6.18°
Hessian determinant	M_6	3.00	0.1	8.10°

for $j = 1,...,6$. As test sequence we take the popular Yosemite sequence *with* clouds. It consists of 15 frames of size 316×252 and combines divergent and translational motion under varying illumination. Both the sequence and its ground truth flow field are available from ftp://csd.uwo.ca under the directory pub/vision. In order to allow for a quantitative comparison of the different data terms we computed the so-called *average angular error (AAE)* as proposed in [9] :

$$\text{AAE}(u_c, u_e) = \frac{1}{|\Omega|} \int_\Omega \arccos\left(\frac{u_c^\top u_e}{|u_c||u_e|}\right) dx. \qquad (18)$$

In this context the subscripts c and e denote the correct respectively the estimated spatiotemporal optic flow vectors $u_c = (u_{c1}, u_{c2}, 1)^\top$ and $u_e = (u_{e1}, u_{e2}, 1)^\top$. Moreover, $|\Omega| = \int_\Omega dx$ is the integration domain, and $|u| = \sqrt{u_1^2 + u_2^2 + 1}$. The obtained results for optimised Gaussian presmoothing parameter σ (cf. equation (1)) and regularsiation parameter α are presented in Table 2. As one can see, the commonly used grey value constancy assumption is outperformed by almost all other constraints that involve higher derivatives. This quantitative impressions are also confirmed qualitatively by the corresponding flow fields shown in Figure 1. While M_1 gives slightly better results at the mountain site, the other data terms are significantly superior in estimating the sky region where illumination changes are present. This shows that it can be worthwhile to replace the brightness constancy constraint by constraints that involve higher derivatives, in particular when varying illumination has to be expected. We also observe that constancy assumptions based on higher order derivatives require a larger Gaussian width σ in order to give optimal results.

3.2 Increasing the Robustness of the Data Term

With M_1–M_6 we have proposed data terms for different illumination conditions and different types of motion. Let us now discuss by the example of M_1 how these data terms can be modified such that they become more robust. To this end we investigate three strategies: local least square fitting, adaptive averaging with nonlinear diffusion, and nonquadratic penalisation.

Local Least Square Fitting A useful strategy to make optic flow estimation more robust under noise is the consideration of neighbourhood information within the data term [26]. To this end one may e.g. assume that the optic flow is constant within some spatial or spatiotemporal neighbourhood of size ρ. Then, simple statistical methods such as least square regressions can be applied to estimate the flow vector from the considered neighbourhood [54]. In this context it is common to decrease the weight of neighbours with increasing distance to the center. Let us now apply such a Gaussian weighted least square fit to $M_1 = u^\top \nabla_3 f \nabla_3 f^\top u$. Then the corresponding data term reads

$$M_7(D^1 f, u) := u^\top J_\rho(\nabla_3 f)\, u \qquad (19)$$

where the *structure tensor* (see e.g. [10, 33, 69])

$$J_\rho(\nabla_3 f) := K_\rho * (\nabla_3 f \nabla_3 f^\top) \qquad (20)$$

results from componentwise Gaussian convolution of the tensor product $J_0 = \nabla_3 f \nabla_3 f^\top$. In this case the standard deviation ρ of the Gaussian K_ρ is called *integration scale*. One should note that for $\rho = 0$ this least square fit by minimising M_7 comes down to the original data term M_1.

Adaptive Averaging with Nonlinear Diffusion Although the preceding integration of local information by means of a Gaussian convolution is a good concept for achieving robustness under noise, the integration relies on the underlying assumption that the optic flow field is constant within the local neighbourhood described by the Gaussian kernel. Especially in the area of discontinuities in the flow field this assumption is not valid, and thus the Gaussian convolution compromises the flow estimation. As a remedy, one can assume that the flow field is only *piecewise* constant. Then one replaces the (linear) structure tensor in (20) that is based on Gaussian convolution – or equivalently linear diffusion – by a nonlinear structure tensor [89, 20] that uses nonlinear tensor-valued diffusion for the local integration. Since nonlinear diffusion reduces the amount of smoothing at discontinuities, it avoids the integration of unrelated data beyond these discontinuities and therefore leads to less ambiguity in the least square regression.

Since the structure tensor is a matrix field, a matrix-valued scheme for nonlinear diffusion is needed. Such a scheme is proposed in [81] where the matrix channels are coupled by a joint diffusivity. With $J_0 = \nabla_3 f \nabla_3 f^\top$ as initial value for the nonlinear diffusion process

$$\partial_t \hat{J}_{ij} = \mathrm{div}\left(g\left(\sum_{k,l=1}^{3} |\nabla \hat{J}_{kl}|^2 \right) \nabla \hat{J}_{ij} \right) \qquad (i,j=1,2,3) \qquad (21)$$

the solution $\hat{J}_t$ constitutes a nonlinear structure tensor for a certain diffusion time t. The diffusion time is the scale parameter of the nonlinear structure tensor, similar to the standard deviation of the Gaussian kernel used in (20), and steers the size of the local neighbourhood. The so-called diffusivity function g is a decreasing function that reduces the amount of smoothing at discontinuities in the data. An appropriate choice is the regularised total variation (TV) diffusivity [5]

$$g(s^2) = \epsilon_1 + \frac{1}{\sqrt{s^2 + \epsilon_2^2}} \tag{22}$$

where the small positive constants ϵ_1 and ϵ_1 are introduced for theoretical reasons and in order to avoid unbounded diffusivities. In practice they can be set, for instance, to 0.001.

If we apply the nonlinear structure tensor to M_1, we obtain the data term

$$M_8(D^1 f, u) := u^\top \hat{J}_t(\nabla_3 f)\, u, \tag{23}$$

which is a nonlinear alternative to M_7.

Alternative ways of creating adaptive structure tensors are studied in [63] and [19]. It is also worth noting that if one chooses the diffusivity function

$$g(s^2) = 1 \tag{24}$$

one ends up with homogeneous diffusion, which does not adapt to the data. Homogeneous diffusion with diffusion time t is equivalent to Gaussian convolution with standard deviation $\rho = \sqrt{2t}$. This shows the direct relation between the employment of the structure tensor J_ρ and the nonlinear structure tensor $\hat{J}_t$.

In our second experiment we compare different data terms regarding their robustness under noise. To this end we have added Gaussian noise with zero mean and varying standard deviation σ_n to the Yosemite sequence *with* clouds. Apart from the data terms M_7 and M_8 that are based on the concept of local integration, we also considered the ordinary data terms M_1 and M_2. As expected, the results in Table 3 show a better performance of the data terms M_7 and M_8 when noise is present. Figure 2 depicts the corresponding flow field for the data term M_7 and $\sigma_n = 40$. Although the original sequence was degraded severely, the computed flow field still looks reasonable. In this context one should also note the worse performance of M_2. It shows that higher-order derivatives are more sensitive to noise.

Nonquadratic Penalisation So far we have only considered data terms that penalise deviations from constancy assumptions in a quadratic way. From a statistical viewpoint, however, it seems desirable to penalise outliers less severely than in a quadratic setting. In particular with regard to the preservation of discontinuities in the data term, this concept from robust statistics [41, 45] proves to be very useful; see e.g. [11, 43, 56]. In order to guarantee well-posedness for the remaining problem and allow the construction of simple globally convergent algorithms it is advantageous to use penalisers $\Psi(s^2)$ that are convex in s. Such penalisers comprise e.g. the regularised TV penaliser [70, 64]

$$\Psi(s^2) = \epsilon_1^2 s^2 + 2\sqrt{s^2 + \epsilon_2^2}, \tag{25}$$

Table 3. Comparison of data terms M_1, M_2, M_7 and M_8 under noise. We added Gaussian noise with varying standard deviations σ_n to the Yosemite sequence with clouds and used a spatial energy functional with homogeneous regularisation to compute the average angular error (AAE). The parameters σ, α, ρ, and t have been optimised.

noise	data term	σ	α	integration parameter	AAE
$\sigma_n = 0$	M_1	1.30	500	-	7.17°
	M_2	2.10	20	-	5.91°
	M_7	1.30	500	$\rho = 1.80$	7.14°
	M_8	1.30	300	$t = 250$	6.97°
$\sigma_n = 20$	M_1	2.08	2200	-	12.17°
	M_2	3.60	35	-	12.26°
	M_7	2.09	1600	$\rho = 10.70$	11.71°
	M_8	2.10	1600	$t = 225$	11.76°
$\sigma_n = 40$	M_1	2.45	4100	-	16.80°
	M_2	4.20	55	-	18.00°
	M_7	2.38	2000	$\rho = 17.60$	15.82°
	M_8	2.40	2500	$t = 500$	16.29°

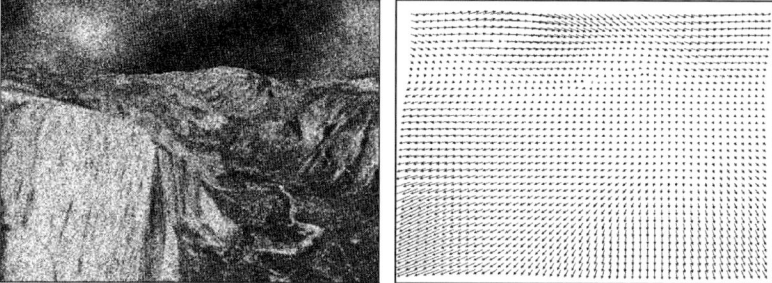

Fig. 2. *(a) Left:* Frame 8 of the Yosemite sequence *with* clouds degraded by Gaussian of standard deviation $\sigma_n = 40$. *(b) Right:* Computed flow field for a spatial approach with data term M_7 (least squares) and homogeneous smoothness term.

where ϵ_1 and ϵ_2 are small positive constants.

In Figure 3 the graphs of the corresponding functions are depicted. Apart from TV penalisation also an example for a nonconvex function is shown. However, one should note that in the case of such nonconvex functions multiple minima have to be expected. As a consequence, minimisation strategies do usually not succeed in finding the global minimum. Let us now replace the quadratic penaliser in M_1 and M_7 by one of the proposed convex functions. Then we obtain the data terms given by

$$M_9(D^1 f, u) := \Psi((u^\top \nabla_3 f)^2),$$
$$M_{10}(D^1 f, u) := \Psi(u^\top J_\rho(\nabla_3 f) u).$$

An overview on the data terms M_7–M_{10} and their capability of handling discontinuities in the data is given in Table 4.

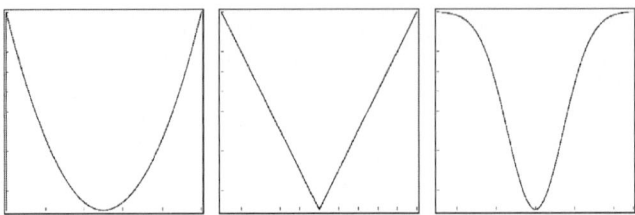

Fig. 3. Comparison of different penalising functions. From left to right: (a) Tikhonov (quadratic). (b) Total variation (linear). (c) Example of a nonconvex function.

Table 4. Comparison of data terms M_7–M_{10} and their suitability for respecting discontinuities in the image sequence.

	data term	concept	discontinuities
M_7	$u^\top J_\rho(\nabla_3 f)\,u$	least squares	no
M_8	$u^\top \tilde{J}_t(\nabla_3 f)\,u$	nonlinear diffusion	yes
M_9	$\Psi((u^\top \nabla_3 f)^2)$	nonquadratic penaliser	yes
M_{10}	$\Psi(u^\top J_\rho(\nabla_3 f)\,u)$	least squares and nonquadratic penaliser	yes

Table 5. Comparison of quadratic and nonquadratic penalisers for the data term M_1 (brightness constancy). We used a spatial energy functional with homogeneous regularisation, and computed the average angular error (AAE) for the Yosemite sequence with clouds. The parameters σ, α and ρ have been optimised.

penaliser	data term	σ	α	ρ	AAE
quadratic	M_1	1.30	500	-	7.17°
nonquadratic	M_9	1.40	190	-	7.08°
nonquadratic + least squares	M_{10}	1.40	200	2.0	6.76°

In our last experiment on the impact of data terms we investigate the advantages of nonquadratic penalisers. This is done in Table 5 where the terms M_1, M_9 and M_{10} are compared. Again, the listed results refer to the Yosemite sequence *with* clouds. Obviously, one can improve the average angular error by replacing the quadratic penaliser with a nonquadratic one. The reason for this improvement can be found in Figure 4. It depicts a zoom into the lower left corner of frame 8 and 9, the ground truth as well as the computed flow fields for the different data terms. As one can see, those boundary pixels from frame 8 that are not present in frame 9 have a large impact on the estimated flow field when penalised in a quadratic way. By using a nonquadratic approach, however, their influence is reduced significantly. As a consequence, the estimation at these locations becomes more precise and the average angular error decreases.

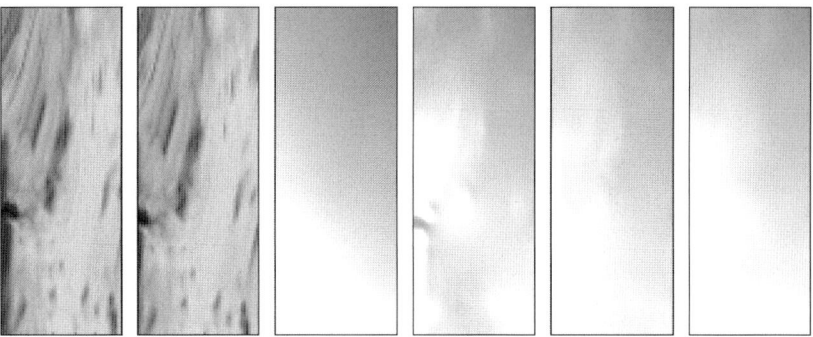

Fig. 4. *From left to right: (a)* Detail from Frame 8 of the Yosemite sequence *with* clouds (48×128 pixels). *(b)* Frame 9. *(c)* Ground truth. *(d)* Computed flow field for a spatial approach with data term M_1 (quadratic penaliser) and homogeneous regularisation. *(e)* Data term M_9 (nonquadratic penaliser). *(f)* Data term M_{10} (nonquadratic penaliser and least squares).

4 Smoothness Terms

So far we have analysed different possibilities for modelling the data term. Let us now explore different models for the smoothness term. This is done in two steps: First we survey a taxonomy that links the regularisers in optic flow functionals to vector-valued diffusion processes. In a second step we investigate the impact of replacing a spatial smoothness assumption by a spatiotemporal one.

4.1 A Diffusion Taxonomy for Smoothness Terms

A taxonomy of the different possibilities to design smoothness constraints has been presented in [91]. It exploits the connection between regularisation methods and diffusion filtering. In order to describe this taxonomy we derive the steepest descent equations for the optic flow functionals. Since they come down to a diffusion–reaction system, we analyse diffusion filters for vector-valued images. Finally we transfer this classification into the optic flow setting.

From Energy Functionals to Diffusion–Reaction Systems Minimising the energy functional (2) can be done in two ways:
One possibility is to compute the so-called Euler–Lagrange equations. They constitute necessary conditions a minimiser of $E(u)$ has to satisfy [29, 36]. In the specific case of a spatial energy functional (2) they are given by the two-dimensional system of partial differential equations (PDEs)

$$0 = \partial_{x_1} S_{u_{1,x_1}} + \partial_{x_2} S_{u_{1,x_2}} - \tfrac{1}{\alpha} \partial_{u_1} M, \qquad (26)$$

$$0 = \partial_{x_1} S_{u_{2,x_1}} + \partial_{x_2} S_{u_{2,x_2}} - \tfrac{1}{\alpha} \partial_{u_2} M \qquad (27)$$

equipped with homogeneous Neumann (reflecting) boundary conditions. The term $S_{u_{i,x_j}}$ denotes the partial derivative of S with respect to $\partial_{x_j} u_i$.

Alternatively we can minimise $E(u)$ by means of the steepest descent method. In the case of a spatial functional we obtain a system of two-dimensional diffusion–reaction equations, where the diffusion term results from the regulariser $S(\nabla f, \nabla u)$, and the reaction term is induced by the data term $M(D^k f, u)$:

$$\partial_t u_1 = \partial_{x_1} S_{u_1,x_1} + \partial_{x_2} S_{u_1,x_2} - \tfrac{1}{\alpha}\partial_{u_1} M, \tag{28}$$

$$\partial_t u_2 = \partial_{x_1} S_{u_2,x_1} + \partial_{x_2} S_{u_2,x_2} - \tfrac{1}{\alpha}\partial_{u_2} M \tag{29}$$

The parameter t is a pure numerical parameter that should not be confused with the time x_3 of the image sequence. If $E(u)$ is strictly convex, a unique minimiser exist and the steepest descent evolution is globally convergent, i.e. its steady–state does not depend on the initialisation. For $t \to \infty$, this steady–state of the diffusion–reaction system is given by the Euler–Lagrange equations (26)–(27).

Since we are interested in a taxonomy for optic flow regularisers, it it sufficient to restrict ourselves to the diffusion part of (28)–(29). This leads to the vector-valued diffusion process

$$\partial_t u_i = \partial_{x_i} S_{u_i,x_1} + \partial_{x_i} S_{u_i,x_2} \qquad (i = 1, 2). \tag{30}$$

In order to get a better understanding of such processes, it is instructive to make a little excursion to diffusion filters for multichannel images. This shall be done next, following the description in [89].

Diffusion of Vector-Valued Images Vector-valued images arise for example as colour images, multispectral satellite images and multi-spin echo MR images. Diffusion filtering of some multichannel image $f = (f_1(x), ..., f_m(x))^\top$ with $x \in \mathbb{R}^2$ may be based on one of the following evolutions:

(a) *Homogeneous diffusion* (introduced in [46] in the scalar case):

$$\partial_t u_i = \Delta u_i \qquad (i = 1, ..., m) \tag{31}$$

(b) *Linear isotropic diffusion* (introduced in [34] in the scalar case):

$$\partial_t u_i = \operatorname{div}\left(g\left(\sum_j |\nabla f_j|^2\right)\nabla u_i\right) \qquad (i = 1, ..., m) \tag{32}$$

(c) *Linear anisotropic diffusion* (introduced in [47] in the scalar case):

$$\partial_t u_i = \operatorname{div}\left(D\left(\sum_j \nabla f_j \nabla f_j^\top\right)\nabla u_i\right) \qquad (i = 1, ..., m) \tag{33}$$

(d) *Nonlinear isotropic diffusion* [37]:

$$\partial_t u_i = \operatorname{div}\left(g\left(\sum_j |\nabla u_j|^2\right)\nabla u_i\right) \qquad (i = 1, ..., m) \tag{34}$$

(e) *Nonlinear anisotropic diffusion [87]:*

$$\partial_t u_i = \mathrm{div}\left(D\left(\sum_j \nabla u_j \nabla u_j^\top\right) \nabla u_i\right) \quad (i=1,...,m) \qquad (35)$$

where $f(x)$ acts as initial condition for the solution $u(x,t)$:

$$u_i(x,0) = f_i(x) \quad (i=1,...,m). \qquad (36)$$

Here, g denotes a scalar-valued diffusivity, and D is a positive definite diffusion matrix. The diffusivity $g(s^2)$ is a decreasing function in its argument. Moreover, we assume that the flux function $g(s^2)s$ is nondecreasing in s. One may e.g. use the regularised TV diffusivity (22). In the *linear* case this ensures that at edges of the *initial* image f, where $\sum_j |\nabla f_j|^2$ is large, the diffusivity $g(\sum_j |\nabla f_j|^2)$ is close to zero. Consequently, diffusion at edges is inhibited. In the *nonlinear* case one introduces a feedback by adapting the diffusivity g to the *evolving* image u. In physics, a diffusion process with a scalar-valued diffusivity is called *isotropic*, since its diffusive behavior does not depend on the direction. Anisotropic diffusion with a direction depending behavior may be realised by replacing the scalar-valued diffusivity g by some positive definite diffusion matrix D. One may design the diffusion matrix D such that diffusion along edges of f or u is preferred and diffusion across edges is inhibited. This may be very useful in cases when noisy edges are present.

How can edge directions in some vector-valued image f be measured? Di Zenzo [30] has proposed to consider the matrix $\sum_j \nabla f_j \nabla f_j^\top$. It serves as a structure tensor for vector-valued images since its eigenvectors v_1, v_2 describe the directions of highest and lowest contrast. This contrast is given by the corresponding eigenvalues μ_1 and μ_2.

A natural choice for the design of some diffusion matrix D as a function of a vector-valued image f would thus be to specify its eigenvectors as the eigenvectors v_1, v_2 of $\sum_j \nabla f_j \nabla f_j^\top$, and its eigenvalues λ_1, λ_2 via

$$\lambda_1 = g(\mu_1), \qquad (37)$$
$$\lambda_2 = g(\mu_2), \qquad (38)$$

with a diffusivity function g as e.g. in (22).
Three remarks are in order here:

1. The fact that in the preceding models the same diffusivity or diffusion matrix is used for all channels ensures that the evolutions between the channels are synchronised. This prevents e.g. that discontinuities evolve at different locations in each channel.
2. Let $J \in \mathbb{R}^{2\times 2}$ be symmetric with eigenvectors v_1, v_2 and eigenvalues μ_1, μ_2:

$$J = \mu_1 v_1 v_1^\top + \mu_2 v_2 v_2^\top. \qquad (39)$$

A formal way to extend some scalar-valued function $g(s^2)$ to a matrix-valued function $g(J)$ is to define

$$g(J) := g(\mu_1)v_1v_1^\top + g(\mu_2)v_2v_2^\top. \tag{40}$$

With this notation we may characterise the linear and nonlinear isotropic models by their diffusivities $g(\sum_j \nabla f_j^\top \nabla f_j)$ and $g(\sum_j \nabla u_j^\top \nabla u_j)$, while their anisotropic counterparts are given by $g(\sum_j \nabla f_j \nabla f_j^\top)$ and $g(\sum_j \nabla u_j \nabla u_j^\top)$. Hence, isotropic and anisotropic models only differ by the location of the transposition.

3. The preceding models are not the only PDE methods that have been proposed for processing vector-valued images. For alternative approaches the reader is referred to [14, 50, 72, 82, 88] and the references therein. Our classification is based on diffusion processes in divergence form that can be derived as steepest descent methods for minimising suitable energy functionals.

Figure L illustrates the effect of the different smoothing strategies for a noisy color image with three channels corresponding to the red, green and blue components. We observe that homogeneous diffusion performs well with respect to denoising, but does not respect image edges. Space-variant linear isotropic diffusion, however, may suffer from noise sensitivity as strong noise may be misinterpreted as an important edge structure where the diffusivity is reduced. Anisotropic linear diffusion allows smoothing along edges, but reduces smoothing across them. This leads to a better performance than isotropic linear diffusion if images are noisy. We can also observe that nonlinear models give better results than their linear counterparts. This is not surprising, since the nonlinear models adapt the diffusion process to the evolving image instead of the initial one.

From Vector-Valued Diffusion to Optic Flow Regularisation Having discussed a taxonomy for vector-valued diffusion, we can transfer it to the optic flow setting. The idea is to identify the optic flow regularisers $S(\nabla f, \nabla u)$ that produce homogeneous, linear isotropic, linear anisotropic, nonlinear isotropic, and nonlinear anisotropic diffusion. It should be noted that now that we returned to the optic flow setting, f denotes the image sequence again, and u is the flow field.

The simplest optic flow regulariser is the *homogeneous* regularisation of Horn and Schunck [44]. This quadratic regulariser of type $S(\nabla u) = |\nabla u_1|^2 + |\nabla u_2|^2$ penalises all deviations from smoothness of the flow field. It can be related to linear diffusion with a constant diffusivity. Thus, the flow field is blurred in a homogeneous way such that motion discontinuities may loose sharpness and get dislocated. It is thus not surprising that people have tried to construct a variety of discontinuity-preserving regularisers. Depending on the structure of the resulting diffusion term, we can classify a regulariser $S(\nabla f, \nabla u)$ as image-driven or flow-driven, and isotropic or anisotropic.

For *image-driven* regularisers, S is not only a function of the flow gradient ∇u but also of the image gradient ∇f. This function is chosen in such a way that it respects discontinuities in the image data. If only the gradient *magnitude* $|\nabla f|$ matters, the method is called *isotropic*. It can avoid smoothing at image edges. An *anisotropic* technique depends also on the *direction* of ∇f. Typically it reduces smoothing across edges of f (i.e. along ∇f), while smoothing along edges of f is still permitted. Image-driven regularisers can be related to linear diffusion processes.

Flow-driven regularisers take into account discontinuities of the unknown flow field u by preventing smoothing at or across flow discontinuities. If the resulting diffusion process uses a scalar-valued diffusivity that only depends on $|\nabla u|^2 := |\nabla u_1|^2 + |\nabla u_2|^2$, it is an *isotropic* process. Cases where also the direction of ∇u_1 and ∇u_2 matters are named *anisotropic*. Flow-driven regularisers lead to nonlinear diffusion processes.

Table 6 gives an overview of the different regularisers and their corresponding diffusion filters. As a rule of thumb, one can expect that flow-driven regularisers offer advantages over image-driven ones for highly textured sequences, where the numerous texture edges create an oversegmentation of the flow field. Moreover, anisotropic methods may give somewhat better results than isotropic ones, since the latter ones are too "lazy" at noisy discontinuities.

Figure 5 presents an experiment that illustrates the impact of the smoothness terms we have discussed so far. We compare the regularisers S_1–S_5 from Table 6 within a spatial approach based on the brightness constancy assumption M_1. In order to illustrate their impact on the flow field, we use the 512×512 *Marble* scene by Otte and Nagel. This sequence that is available at http://i21www.ira.uka.de/image-sequences consists of 31 frames and requires the estimation of flow discontinuities within a globally translational motion. Figure 5 depicts a zoom into the computed flow fields, where one of these discontinuities is shown. The performance of the different regularisers is not surprising: Homogeneous regularisation is fairly blurry and cannot preserve the discontinuity. Flow-driven and image-driven regularisers perform better whereby the usage of flow information offers advantages in textured regions. And finally, one observes that anisotropic regularisation yields slightly more accurate results than the isotropic one.

4.2 Spatiotemporal Regularisation

While our general functional (2) allows either spatial or spatiotemporal models, the regularisers that we have discussed so far use only *spatial* smoothness constraints. Thus, it would be natural to impose some amount of (piecewise) *temporal* smoothness as well. Let us now investigate what happens if we consider such spatiotemporal models.

Going from spatial to spatiotemporal models is not very difficult in principle: All one has to do is to replace the spatial integration domain Ω in (2) by a spatiotemporal one, and to consider spatiotemporal instead of spatial derivatives. As a resulting steepest descent method, one obtains the three-dimensional diffusion–reaction system

$$\partial_t u_1 = \partial_{x_1} S_{u_{1,x_1}} + \partial_{x_2} S_{u_{1,x_2}} + \partial_{x_3} S_{u_{1,x_3}} - \tfrac{1}{\alpha} \partial_{u_1} M, \tag{41}$$

$$\partial_t u_2 = \partial_{x_1} S_{u_{2,x_1}} + \partial_{x_2} S_{u_{2,x_2}} + \partial_{x_3} S_{u_{2,x_3}} - \tfrac{1}{\alpha} \partial_{u_2} M \tag{42}$$

instead of its two-dimensional counterpart (28)–(29).

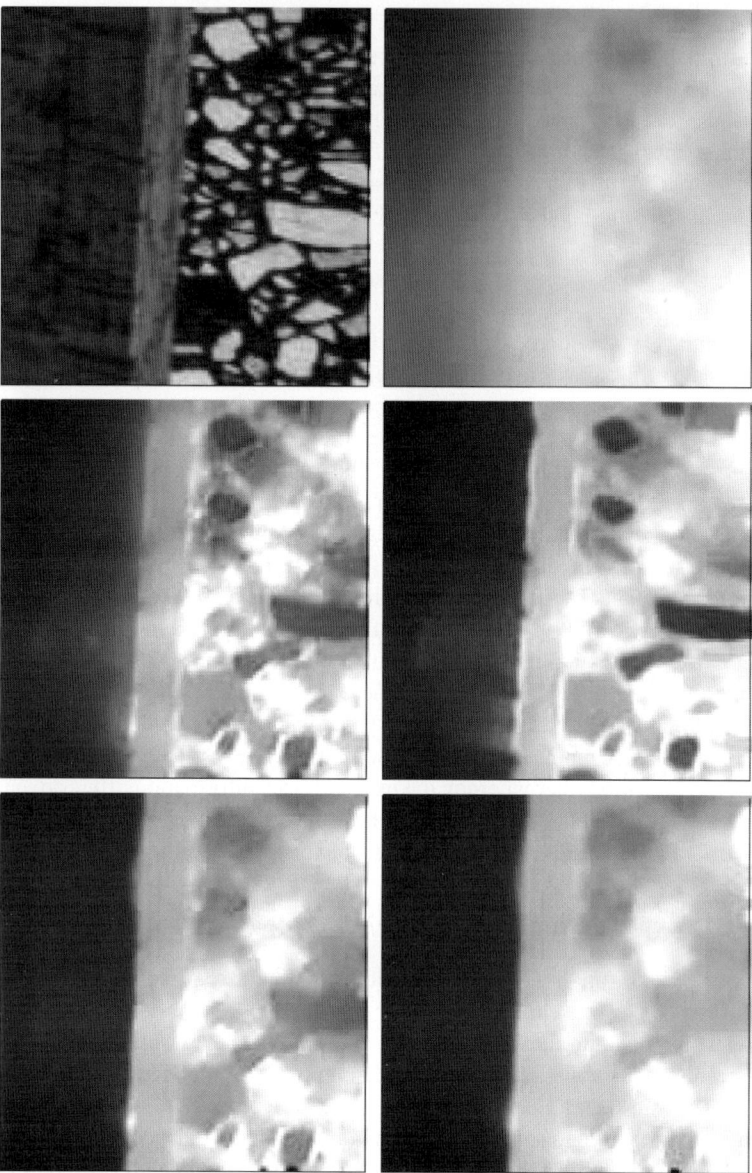

Fig. 5. *(a) Top left:* Detail from Frame 16 of the *Marble* sequence (128×128 pixels). *(b) Top right:* Computed optic flow magnitude for a spatial approach with data term M_1 (brightness constancy) and smoothness term S_1 (homogeneous regularisation). *(c) Middle left:* Smoothness term S_2 (image-driven isotropic regularisation). *(d) Middle right:* Smoothness term S_3 (image-driven anisotropic regularisation). *(e) Bottom left:* Smoothness term S_4 (flow-driven isotropic regularisation) *(f) Bottom right:* Smoothness term S_5 (flow-driven anisotropic regularisation). From [91].

Table 6. Vector-valued diffusion processes and their corresponding optic flow regularisers. In the diffusion context, f denotes the vector-valued initial image and u its evolution. In the optic flow setting, f is the scalar-valued image sequence and u describes the optic flow field.

vector-valued diffusion process $\partial_t u_i = \partial_{x_1} S_{u_{i x_1}} + \partial_{x_2} S_{u_{i x_2}}$	optic flow regulariser $S(\nabla f, \nabla u)$
homogeneous $\partial_t u_i = \Delta u_i$ (scalar case: Iijima 1959 [46])	homogeneous $S_1 = \sum_{i=1}^{2} \|\nabla u_i\|^2$ (Horn/Schunck 1981 [44])
linear isotropic $\partial_t u_i = \mathrm{div}\left(g(\sum_j \|\nabla f_j\|^2)\, \nabla u_i\right)$ (scalar case: Fritsch 1992 [34])	image-driven, isotropic $S_2 = g(\|\nabla f\|^2) \sum_{i=1}^{2} \|\nabla u_i\|^2$ (Alvarez et al. 1999 [2])
linear anisotropic $\partial_t u_i = \mathrm{div}\left(g(\sum_j \nabla f_j \nabla f_j^\top)\, \nabla u_i\right)$ (scalar case: Iijima 1962 [47])	image-driven, anisotropic $S_3 = \sum_{i=1}^{2} \nabla u_i^\top D(\nabla f) \nabla u_i$ (Nagel 1983 [60])
nonlinear isotropic $\partial_t u_i = \mathrm{div}\left(\Psi'(\sum_j \|\nabla u_j\|^2)\, \nabla u_i\right)$ (Gerig et al. 1992 [37])	flow-driven, isotropic $S_4 = \Psi\left(\sum_{i=1}^{2} \|\nabla u_i\|^2\right)$ (Schnörr 1994 [73])
nonlinear anisotropic $\partial_t u_i = \mathrm{div}\left(\Psi'(\sum_j \nabla u_j \nabla u_j^\top)\, \nabla u_i\right)$ (Weickert 1994 [87])	flow-driven, anisotropic $S_5 = \mathrm{trace}\,\Psi\left(\sum_{i=1}^{2} \nabla u_i \nabla u_i^\top\right)$ (Weickert/Schnörr 2001 [91])

In practice, spatiotemporal models have not been used too often so far. An early suggestion for spatiotemporal anisotropic image-driven regularisers goes back to Nagel [61], followed by spatiotemporal flow-driven approaches such as [11, 92]. It appears that the limited memory of previous computer architectures prevented many researchers from studying approaches with spatiotemporal regularisers, since they require to keep the entire image stack in the computer memory. On contemporary PCs, however, these memory requirements are no longer a severe restriction in most cases. With respect to the computing time, the additional requirements are moderate if the entire sequence has to be analysed anyway. Often spatiotemporal models reward their users by significantly improved optic flow estimates. It is thus likely that spatiotemporal regularisers will become more important in the future.

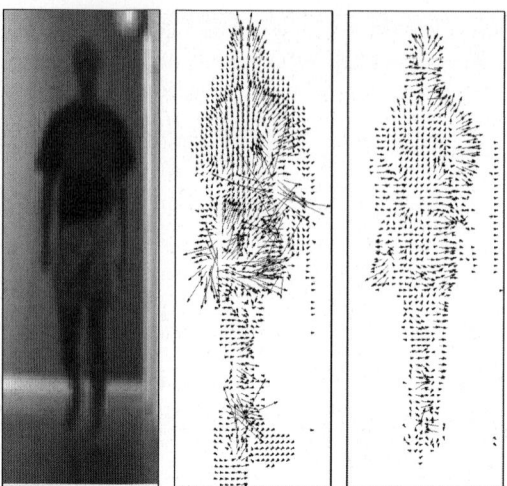

Fig. 6. *(a) Left:* Detail of Frame 8 of the *Copenhagen hallway* sequence. *(b) Middle:* Computed flow field for the spatial approach with data term M_1 (brightness constancy) and smoothness term S_4 (isotropic flow-driven regularisation). *(c) Right:* Ditto for the spatiotemporal approach. From [92].

In Figure 6 we study the effect of replacing spatial by spatiotemporal regularisation. This is done by the example of the 256×256 *Copenhagen hallway* sequence by Olsen and Nielsen. This real-world sequence consists of 16 frames and shows a person who walks along a hallway towards the camera. Comparing the quality of both flow fields, one sees that the additional assumption of temporal smoothness may lead to significantly improved results. In particular the displacements of fast moving body parts such as arms and legs are estimated with a much higher precision.

5 Experiments with Suitable Combinations

In the previous experiments we have focused either on the data or on the smoothness term. Let us now present experiments that illustrate how useful suitable combinations of these terms are.

We start by considering a spatial approach with the least square regression data term M_7 and homogeneous regulariser S_1. Then we replace the quadratic penalisers in *both* the data and the smoothness term by nonquadratic penalising functions. Thus, a spatial approach with data term M_{10} and isotropic flow-driven regulariser S_4 is obtained. And finally, the energy functionals of both the original and the modified variant are extended to the spatiotemporal domain.

A comparison of these four approaches is performed in Table 7 where average angular errors for the *Marble* sequence are listed. The improvements of the results thereby clearly show that established concepts in data and smoothness term should

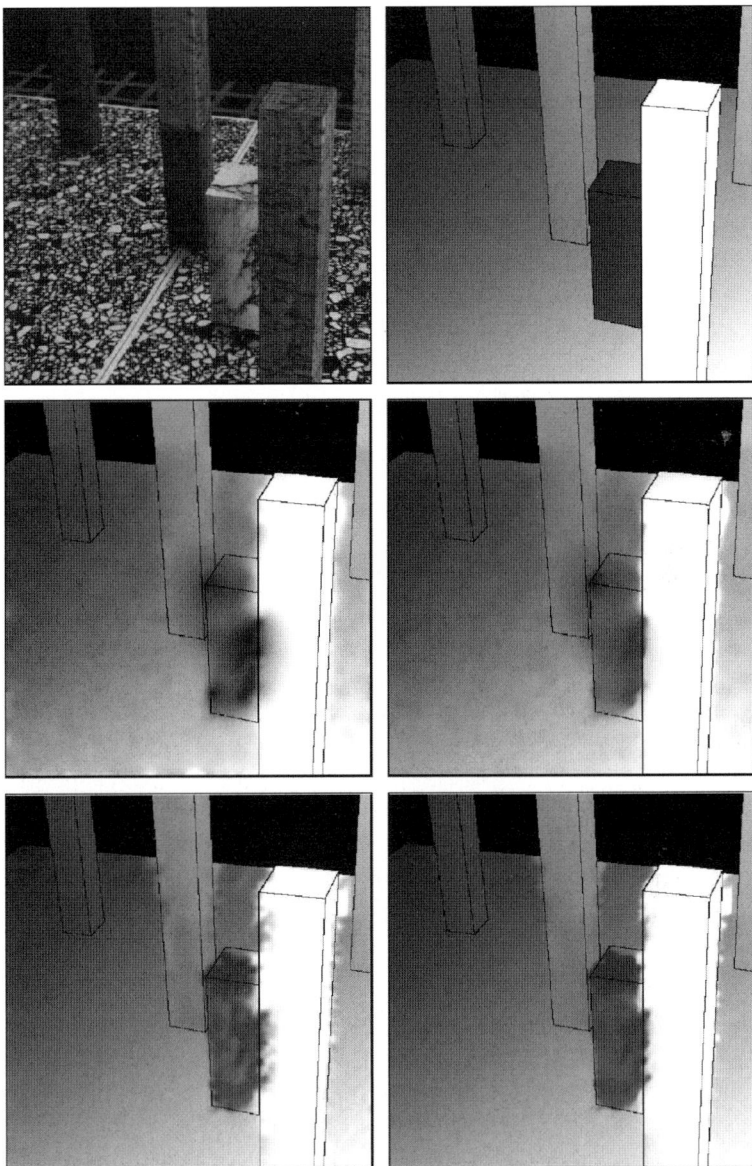

Fig. 7. *(a) Top left:* Frame 16 of the *Marble* sequence. *(b) Top right:* Ground truth magnitude. *(c) Middle left:* Computed flow field for a spatial approach with data term M_7 (least squares) and smoothness term S_1 (homogeneous regularisation). *(d) Middle right:* Ditto with data term M_{10} (nonquadratic and least squares) and smoothness term S_4 (isotropic flow-driven regularisation). *(e) Bottom left:* Spatiotemporal approach with data term M_7 (least squares) and smoothness term S_1 (homogeneous regularisation). *(f) Bottom right:* Ditto with data term M_{10} (nonquadratic and least squares) and smoothness term S_4 (isotropic flow-driven regularisation). Adapted from [26].

Table 7. Results for different combinations based on local integration. The average angular error (AAE) has been computed for the *Marble* sequence. Adapted from [26].

approach	data term	smoothness term	AAE
2-D quadratic	M_7	S_1	5.30°
2-D nonquadratic	M_{10}	S_4	5.14°
3-D quadratic	M_7	S_1	2.06°
3-D nonquadratic	M_{10}	S_4	1.70°

be combined in order to obtain the best performance. This is also confirmed by Figure 7, where we depict the computed flow fields. One can see that each component contributes to the overall improvement: The non-quadratic data term improves the estimation for outliers in the boundary region, the flow-driven isotropic regulariser allows a better preservation of the discontinuities at the marbled blocks and the temporal extension produces a more homogeneous estimation of the floor.

In a second experiment we replace the brightness constancy assumption within M_{10} by the gradient constancy assumption used in M_2. Let us denote this new data term by M_{11}. In Table 8 the resulting spatial and spatiotemporal approach are compared to other methods from the literature, when being applied to the Yosemite sequence with clouds. With 2.78° respectively 3.50° very low average angular errors are obtained[1]. The corresponding flow fields for the spatiotemporal method are depicted in Fig. 8. Obviously, they match the ground truth very well. This shows that sophisticated variational approaches belong to the qualitatively best performing optic flow methods.

6 Well-Posedness Results

One specific advantage of convex variational methods for optic flow computations results from the fact that they allow a rigorous mathematical analysis. As an example, the following result has been proven in [91] for spatial or spatiotemporal energy functionals with the brightness constancy assumption as data term M_1 and any of the smoothness terms $S_1,...,S_5$:

Theorem (Well-Posedness of Optic Flow Functionals).
Assume that the following properties hold:

(a) The penalising function $\Psi(s^2)$ is differentiable and strictly convex in $s \in \mathbb{R}$.
(b) There exist $c_1, c_2 > 0$ such that $c_1 s^2 \leq \Psi(s^2) \leq c_2 s^2$ for all s.
(c) The initial data are sufficiently smooth: $f \in H^1(\Omega)$.
(d) f_{x_1} and f_{x_2} are linearly independent in $L^2(\Omega)$ and have finite $L^\infty(\Omega)$ norm.

Then the (spatial or spatiotemporal) energy functional

---

[1]This method has been further modified in [18] where it yielded the best results in the literature so far.

Table 8. Comparison between results from the literature with 100 % density and our results using a 3-D functional with data term M_{11} (nonquadratic penalised gradient constancy) and smoothness term S_4 (isotropic flow-driven regulariser). All data refer to the *Yosemite* sequence with cloudy sky. Multiscale means that some focusing strategy using linear scale-space or pyramids has been applied. AAE = average angular error.

technique	multiscale	AAE
Horn/Schunck, original [9]	no	31.69°
Singh, step 1 [9]	no	15.28°
Anandan [9]	no	13.36°
Singh, step 2 [9]	no	10.44°
Nagel [9]	no	10.22°
Horn/Schunck, modified [9]	no	9.78°
Uras *et al.*, unthresholded [9]	no	8.94°
Alvarez/Weickert/Sánchez [3]	yes	5.53°
Mémin/Pérez (IEEE TIP) [56]	yes	5.38°
Bruhn/Weickert/Schnörr [26]	no	5.18°
Mémin/Pérez (ICCV '98) [57]	yes	4.69°
2-D nonquadratic / gradient constancy ($M_{11} + S_4$)	**no**	**3.50°**
3-D nonquadratic / gradient constancy ($M_{11} + S_4$)	**no**	**2.78°**

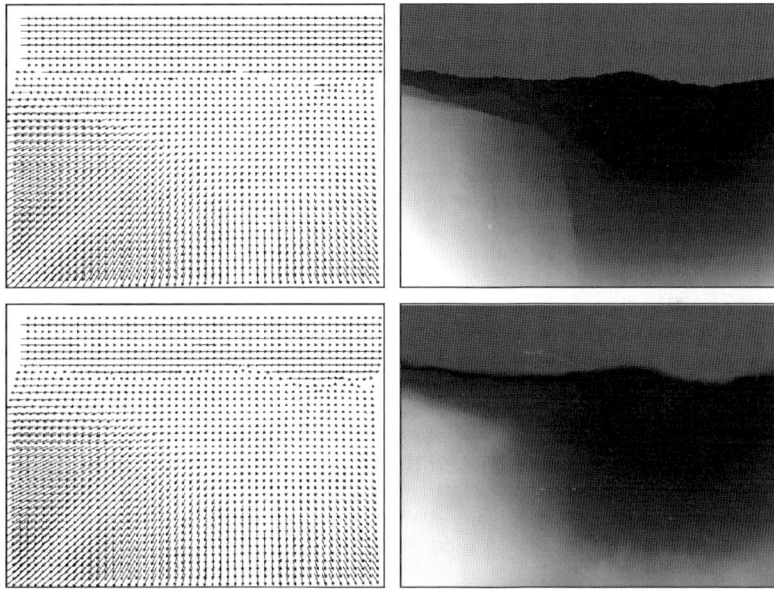

Fig. 8. *(a) Top left:* Ground truth for the Yosemite sequence *with* clouds. *(b) Top right:* Magnitude of the ground truth. *(c) Bottom left:* Computed flow field for a spatiotemporal approach with data term M_{11} (nonquadratic gradient constancy) and smoothness term S_4 (isotropic flow-driven regularisation). *(d) Bottom right:* Magnitude of the computed flow field.

$$E(u) = \int_\Omega \left(\langle u, \nabla_3 f \rangle^2 + \alpha\, S_j(\nabla f, \nabla u) \right) dx \qquad (43)$$

with $j \in \{1,...,5\}$ has a unique minimiser $w := (u_1, u_2) \in H^1(\Omega) \times H^1(\Omega) =: \mathcal{H}$. It depends in a continuous way on the image sequence f.

The proof of this theorem combines methods from [75] and from [91] where two essential properties are required:

1. In order to guarantee strict convexity of the smoothness term, a convexity estimate for matrices is needed:
   Let $\Psi: \mathbb{R} \to \mathbb{R}$ be strictly convex, A and B two positive semidefinite symmetric $m \times m$ matrices with $A \neq B$, and $\beta \in (0,1)$. Then

$$\operatorname{trace} \Psi(\beta A + (1-\beta) B) < \beta \operatorname{trace} \Psi(A) + (1-\beta) \operatorname{trace} \Psi(B). \qquad (44)$$

2. On the other hand, strict convexity of the data term requires to address degeneracies by showing that there exists a constant $c > 0$ such that

$$\int_\Omega \left((\nabla f^\top w)^2 + \gamma |\nabla w|^2 \right) dx \geq c \|w\|_\mathcal{H}^2, \qquad \forall w \in \mathcal{H}. \qquad (45)$$

It should be noted that such a well-posedness proof is much more than a pure theoretical result: In practise it also guarantees e.g. stability of the optic flow field with respect to noise that perturbs the image data. In this sense it is the real reason behind the high robustness that distinguishes good variational approaches from a number of alternative ways to estimate the optic flow field. For alternative ways to obtain well-posedness results for optic flow functionals we refer to [6, 7, 43].

7 Algorithms

For the numerical minimisation of the energy functional (2), two strategies are used very frequently:

In the first strategy, one discretises the parabolic diffusion–reaction system (28), (29) and recovers the optic flow field as the steady–state solution for $t \to \infty$. The simplest numerical scheme would be an explicit (Euler forward) finite difference scheme [58, 59, 76]. More efficient methods include semi-implicit approaches that offer better stability properties at the expense of the need to solve linear systems of equations.

Alternatively, one can directly discretise the elliptic Euler-Lagrange equations (26), (27), either by finite differences [58, 59, 76] or finite elements [27, 85]. This also requires to solve large linear or nonlinear systems of equations. Efficient methods for this task include *successive overrelaxation (SOR)* methods [84, 94], *preconditioned conjugate gradient (PCG)* algorithms [55, 71] and *multigrid* techniques [16, 17, 40, 80, 93].

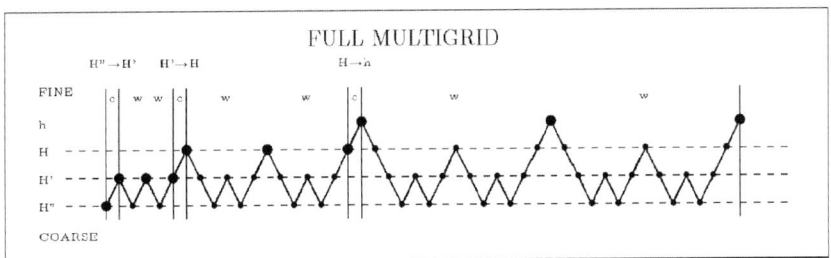

Fig. 9. Example of a full multigrid implementation for four levels. Starting from a coarse scale the solution is refined step by step. From [22].

Table 9. Performance benchmark for the 316×252 Yosemite sequence with clouds. FPS = frames per second. Runtimes refer to the computation of all 14 frames with a numerical precision of 10^{-3}. The implementation was done in C on a 3.06 GHz Pentium 4 PC. The obtained average angular error is $7.17°$. From [22].

solver	iterations/frame	runtime [s]	FPS [s^{-1}]	speedup
Gauß–Seidel	21931	543.799	0.026	1
SOR	286	10.140	1.381	54
Gauß–Seidel, coarse-to-fine	237	8.399	1.667	65
SOR, coarse-to-fine	25	1.723	8.125	316
full multigrid	1	0.768	18.229	708

Figure 9 illustrates an example of a full multigrid cycle with 4 levels. Such strategies have been used in [22, 23] for finding the minimum of a variational approach with data term M_2 and a homogeneous regulariser. Thus, it was possible to compute up to 18 dense flow fields of size 316×252 pixels on 3.06 GHz Pentium 4 PC within a single second. Table 9 compares the performance of this numerical scheme to widely used iterative solvers like the Gauß-Seidel method or its extrapolated SOR variant. As one can see, the full multigrid cycle is almost three orders of magnitude more efficient than the Gauß-Seidel relaxation scheme and 13 times faster than the SOR method. Even frequently used coarse-to-fine strategies without error correction steps are outperformed clearly. This shows that computational efficiency is no problem for variational optic flow methods, when state-of-the-art numerical methods are used.

While this example refers to a quadratic energy functional that leads to linear Euler–Lagrange equations, it is also possible to achieve real-time performance with nonquadratic functionals that give rise to nonlinear Euler–Lagrange equations. This is shown in [24] as well as in [25] where a larger variety of methods is studied.

8 A Simple and General Confidence Measure

While global, energy-based optic flow methods yield dense flow fields due to the filling-in effect, it is clear that the flow estimates cannot have the same reliability at all locations. It would thus be interesting to find a confidence measure that allows to assess the reliability of a dense optic flow field. In 1994 Barron *et al.* [9] have identified the absence of such good measure as one of the main drawbacks of energy-based global optic flow techniques: Simple heuristics such as using $|\nabla f|$ as a confidence measure did not work well. As a remedy, we present a confidence measure that is not only very simple, but also suited for any variational optic flow method. In our description we follow [26].

Since the energy functional E penalises deviations from model assumptions by summing up the deviations E_i from all pixels i in the image domain, it appears natural to use E_i for assessing the local reliability of the computation. All we have to do is to consider the cumulative histogram of the contributions E_i of all pixels $i \in \{1,...,N\}$ in the image domain. As an approximation to the p percent locations with the highest reliability, we look for the p percent locations where the contribution E_i is lowest. There are very efficient algorithms available for this purpose; see e.g. [67, Section 8.5].

Let us now evaluate the quality of our energy-based confidence measure. To this end we consider the spatiotemporal energy functional with the local least square fit data term M_7 and the isotropic flow-driven regulariser S_4. In [26], this technique is named *3-D CLG (combined local–global) method*. Figure 10(a) depicts the 20 % quantile of locations where the 3-D CLG method has lowest contributions to the energy. A comparison with Figure 10(b) – which displays the result of a theoretical confidence measure that would be optimal with respect to the average angular error – demonstrates that the energy-based confidence method leads to a fairly realistic sparsification of flow fields. In particular, we observe that this confidence criterion is very successful in removing the cloudy sky regions. These locations are well-known to create large angular errors in many optic flow methods [9]. A number of authors have thus only used the modified *Yosemite* sequence without cloudy sky, or they have neglected the flow values from the sky region for their evaluations

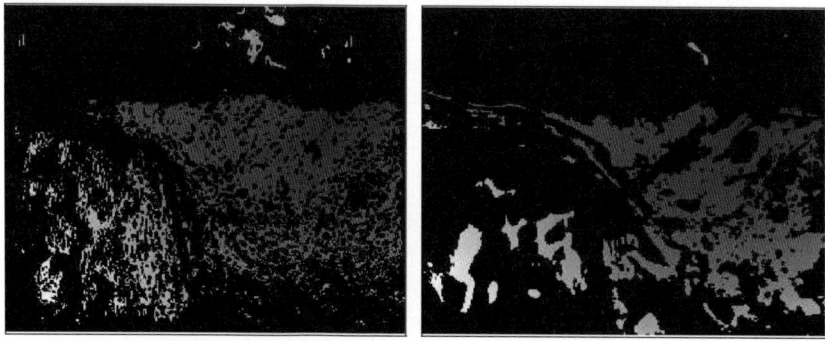

Fig. 10. Confidence criterion for the *Yosemite* sequence with clouds. *(a) Left:* Locations with the lowest contributions to the energy (20 % quantile). The non-black grey values depict the optic flow magnitude. *(b) Right:* Locations where the angular error is lowest (20 % quantile).

[8, 12, 13, 31, 32, 48, 49, 53, 77]. As we have seen one may get significantly lower angular errors than for the full sequence with cloudy sky.

A quantitative evaluation of our confidence measure is given in Table 10. Here we have used the energy-based confidence measure to sparsify the dense flow field such that the reduced density coincides with densities of well-known optic flow methods. Most of them have been evaluated by Barron et al. [9]. We observe that the sparsified 3-D CLG method performs very favourably: It has a far lower angular error than all corresponding methods with the same density. In several cases there is an order of magnitude between these approaches. At a flow density of 2.4 %, an average angular error of 0.76 ° is reached. To our knowledge, these are the best values that have been obtained for this sequence in the entire literature. It should be noted that these results have been computed from an image sequence that suffers from quantisation errors since its grey values have been stored in 8-bit precision only.

In Table 10 we also observe that the angular error decreases *monotonically* under sparsification over the entire range from 100 % down to 2.4 %. This in turn indicates an interesting finding that may seem counterintuitive at first glance: *Regions in which the filling-in effect dominates give particularly small angular errors.* In such flat regions, the data term vanishes such that a smoothly extended flow field may yield only a small local contribution to the energy functional. If there were

Table 10. Comparison between the "nondense" results from Barron et al. [9], Weber and Malik [86], Ong and Spann [66] and our results for the *Yosemite* sequence with cloudy sky. AAE = average angular error. CLG = average angular error of the 3-D CLG method with the same density. The sparse flow field has been created using our energy-based confidence criterion. The table shows that using this criterion clearly outperforms all results in the evaluation of Barron et al.

Technique	Density	AAE	CLG
Singh, step 2, $\lambda_1 \leq 0.1$	97.7 %	10.03°	6.04°
Ong/Spann	89.9 %	5.76°	5.26°
Heeger, level 0	64.2 %	22.82°	3.00°
Weber/Malik	64.2 %	4.31°	3.00°
Horn/Schunck, original, $|\nabla f| \geq 5$	59.6 %	25.33°	2.72°
Ong/Spann, tresholded	58.4 %	4.16°	2.66°
Heeger, combined	44.8 %	15.93°	2.07°
Lucas/Kanade, $\lambda_2 \geq 1.0$	35.1 %	4.28°	1.71°
Fleet/Jepson, $\tau = 2.5$	34.1 %	4.63°	1.67°
Horn/Schunck, modified, $|\nabla f| \geq 5$	32.9 %	5.59°	1.63°
Nagel, $|\nabla f| \geq 5$	32.9 %	6.06°	1.63°
Fleet/Jepson, $\tau = 1.25$	30.6 %	5.28°	1.55°
Heeger, level 1	15.2 %	9.87°	1.15°
Uras et al., $\det(H) \geq 1$	14.7 %	7.55°	1.14°
Singh, step 1, $\lambda_1 \leq 6.5$	11.3 %	12.01°	1.07°
Waxman et al., $\sigma_f = 2.0$	7.4 %	20.05°	0.95°
Heeger, level 2	2.4 %	12.93°	0.76°

large angular errors in regions with such low energy contributions, our confidence measure would not work well for low densities. This also confirms the observation that $|\nabla f|$ is not necessarily a good confidence measure [9]: Areas with large gradients may represent noise or occlusions, where reliable flow information is difficult to obtain. The filling-in effect, however, may create more reliable information in flat regions by averaging less reliable information that comes from all the surrounding high-gradient regions. A more extensive experimental evaluation of the energy based confidence measure is presented in [21].

9 Summary and Extensions

In this chapter we have outlined some basic design principles for variational optic flow methods and studied their performance in a number of experiments. For theoretical and practical reasons we have restricted ourselves to convex energy functionals that use linearised data terms. They are valid approximations when the temporal sampling is sufficiently fine such that the displacements between subsequent frames are small. We have seen that contemporary variational optic flow models have reached a high degree of sophistication that allows to achieve highly accurate computations of the displacement fields. Moreover, they are mathematically well-founded, they allow real-time computations on standard hardware, and it is possible to apply a simple and intuitive confidence measure.

There are several possibilities to improve the performance of these methods even further: One may for instance use data terms that renounce linearisations [3, 11, 62]. They create models that are better suitable for large displacements between subsequent frames. Unfortunately they lead to nonconvex functionals that may possess numerous local minimisres. In such a case one often uses multilevel strategies that encourage convergence towards a global minimiser [3, 4, 56]. Another extension that becomes relevant for large displacements consists of using modified functionals in order to deal with occlusion problems [1, 68]. On the numerical side, parallelisation strategies can be investigated, e.g. domain decomposition methods [51]. A detailed discussion of these extensions is beyond the scope of the present chapter.

It is our hope that the models we have described do not remain restricted to optic flow computation, but will also prove their use in related correspondence problems such as stereo reconstruction and image registration.

Acknowledgements. Our research has partly been funded by the *Deutsche Forschungsgemeinschaft (DFG)* and the *Graduiertenkolleg "Leistungsgarantien für Rechnersysteme"*. This is gratefully acknowledged.

References

1. L. Alvarez, R. Deriche, T. Papadopoulo, and J. Sánchez. Symmetrical dense optical flow estimation with occlusion detection. In A. Heyden, G. Sparr, M. Nielsen, and P. Jo-

hansen, editors, *Computer Vision – ECCV 2002*, volume 2350 of *Lecture Notes in Computer Science*, pages 721–736. Springer, Berlin, 2002.
2. L. Alvarez, J. Esclarín, M. Lefébure, and J. Sánchez. A PDE model for computing the optical flow. In *Proc. XVI Congreso de Ecuaciones Diferenciales y Aplicaciones*, pages 1349–1356, Las Palmas de Gran Canaria, Spain, September 1999.
3. L. Alvarez, J. Weickert, and J. Sánchez. Reliable estimation of dense optical flow fields with large displacements. *International Journal of Computer Vision*, 39(1):41–56, August 2000.
4. P. Anandan. A computational framework and an algorithm for the measurement of visual motion. *International Journal of Computer Vision*, 2:283–310, 1989.
5. F. Andreu–Vaillo, V. Caselles, and J. M. Mazon. *Parabolic Quasilinaer Equations Minimizing Linear Growth Functionals*, volume 223 of *Progress in Mathematics*. Birkhäuser, Basel, 2004.
6. G. Aubert, R. Deriche, and P. Kornprobst. Computing optical flow via variational techniques. *SIAM Journal on Applied Mathematics*, 60(1):156–182, 1999.
7. G. Aubert and P. Kornprobst. *Mathematical Problems in Image Processing: Partial Differential Equations and the Calculus of Variations*, volume 147 of *Applied Mathematical Sciences*. Springer, New York, 2002.
8. A. Bab-Hadiashar and D. Suter. Robust optic flow computation. *International Journal of Computer Vision*, 29(1):59–77, August 1998.
9. J. L. Barron, D. J. Fleet, and S. S. Beauchemin. Performance of optical flow techniques. *International Journal of Computer Vision*, 12(1):43–77, February 1994.
10. J. Bigün, G. H. Granlund, and J. Wiklund. Multidimensional orientation estimation with applications to texture analysis and optical flow. *IEEE Transactions on Pattern Analysis and Machine Intelligence*, 13(8):775–790, August 1991.
11. M. J. Black and P. Anandan. Robust dynamic motion estimation over time. In *Proc. 1991 IEEE Computer Society Conference on Computer Vision and Pattern Recognition*, pages 292–302, Maui, HI, June 1991. IEEE Computer Society Press.
12. M. J. Black and P. Anandan. The robust estimation of multiple motions: parametric and piecewise smooth flow fields. *Computer Vision and Image Understanding*, 63(1):75–104, January 1996.
13. M. J. Black and A. Jepson. Estimating optical flow in segmented images using variable-order parametric models with local deformations. *IEEE Transactions on Pattern Analysis and Machine Intelligence*, 18(10):972–986, October 1996.
14. P. Blomgren and T. F. Chan. Color TV: total variation methods for restoration of vector valued images. *IEEE Transactions on Image Processing*, 7(3):304–309, March 1998.
15. A. Borzi, K. Ito, and K. Kunisch. Optimal control formulation for determining optical flow. *SIAM Journal on Scientific Computing*, 24(3):818–847, 2002.
16. A. Brandt. Multi-level adaptive solutions to boundary-value problems. *Mathematics of Computation*, 31(138):333–390, April 1977.
17. W. L. Briggs, V. E. Henson, and S. F. McCormick. *A Multigrid Tutorial*. SIAM, Philadelphia, second edition, 2000.
18. T. Brox, A. Bruhn, N. Papenberg, and J. Weickert. High accuracy optical flow estimation based on a theory for warping. In T. Pajdla and J. Matas, editors, *Computer Vision – ECCV 2004, Part IV*, volume 3024 of *Lecture Notes in Computer Science*, pages 25–36. Springer, Berlin, 2004.
19. T. Brox, R. van den Boomgaard, F. Lauze, J. van de Weijer, J. Weickert, R. Mrázek, and P. Kornprobst. Adaptive structure tensors and their applications. In J. Weickert and H. Hagen, editors, *Visualization and Image Processing of Tensor Fields*. Springer, Berlin, 2005. To appear.

20. T. Brox and J. Weickert. Nonlinear matrix diffusion for optic flow estimation. In L. Van Gool, editor, *Pattern Recognition*, volume 2449 of *Lecture Notes in Computer Science*, pages 446–453. Springer, Berlin, 2002.
21. A. Bruhn and J. Weickert. Confidence measures for variational optic flow methods. In R. Klette, R. Kozera, L. Noakes, and J. Weickert, editors, *Geometric Properties from Incomplete Data*, Computational Imaging and Vision. Springer, Dordrecht, 2005. To appear.
22. A. Bruhn, J. Weickert, C. Feddern, T. Kohlberger, and C. Schnörr. Real-time optic flow computation with variational methods. In N. Petkov and M. A. Westenberg, editors, *Computer Analysis of Images and Patterns*, volume 2756 of *Lecture Notes in Computer Science*, pages 222–229. Springer, Berlin, 2003.
23. A. Bruhn, J. Weickert, C. Feddern, T. Kohlberger, and C. Schnörr. Variational optic flow computation in real-time. *IEEE Transactions on Image Processing*, 14(5):608–615, May 2005.
24. A. Bruhn, J. Weickert, T. Kohlberger, and C. Schnörr. Discontinuity-preserving computation of variational optic flow in real-time. In R. Kimmel, N. Sochen, and J. Weickert, editors, *Scale-Space and PDE Methods in Computer Vision*, volume 3459 of *Lecture Notes in Computer Science*, pages 585–597, Berlin, 2005. Springer.
25. A. Bruhn, J. Weickert, T. Kohlberger, and C. Schnörr. A multigrid platform for real-time motion computation with discontinuity-preserving variational methods. Technical report, Dept. of Mathematics, Saarland University, Saarbrücken, Germany, May 2005. Submitted to *International Journal of Computer Vision*.
26. A. Bruhn, J. Weickert, and C. Schnörr. Lucas/Kanade meets Horn/Schunck: Combining local and global optic flow methods. *International Journal of Computer Vision*, 61(3):211–231, 2005.
27. P. G. Ciarlet. *The Finite Element Method for Elliptic Problems*. SIAM, Philadelphia, 2002.
28. I. Cohen. Nonlinear variational method for optical flow computation. In *Proc. Eighth Scandinavian Conference on Image Analysis*, volume 1, pages 523–530, Tromsø, Norway, May 1993.
29. R. Courant and D. Hilbert. *Methods of Mathematical Physics*, volume 1. Interscience, New York, 1953.
30. S. Di Zenzo. A note on the gradient of a multi-image. *Computer Vision, Graphics and Image Processing*, 33:116–125, 1986.
31. G. Farnebäck. Fast and accurate motion estimation using orientation tensors and parametric motion models. In *Proc. 15th International Conference on Pattern Recognition*, volume 1, pages 135–139, Barcelona, Spain, September 2000.
32. G. Farnebäck. Very high accuracy velocity estimation using orientation tensors, parametric motion, and simultaneous segmentation of the motion field. In *Proc. Eighth International Conference on Computer Vision*, volume 1, pages 171–177, Vancouver, Canada, July 2001. IEEE Computer Society Press.
33. W. Förstner and E. Gülch. A fast operator for detection and precise location of distinct points, corners and centres of circular features. In *Proc. ISPRS Intercommission Conference on Fast Processing of Photogrammetric Data*, pages 281–305, Interlaken, Switzerland, June 1987.
34. D. S. Fritsch. A medial description of greyscale image structure by gradient-limited diffusion. In R. A. Robb, editor, *Visualization in Biomedical Computing '92*, volume 1808 of *Proceedings of SPIE*, pages 105–117. SPIE Press, Bellingham, 1992.

35. B. Galvin, B. McCane, K. Novins, D. Mason, and S. Mills. Recovering motion fields: an analysis of eight optical flow algorithms. In *Proc. 1998 British Machine Vision Conference*, Southampton, England, September 1998.
36. I. M. Gelfand and S. V. Fomin. *Calculus of Variations*. Dover, New York, 2000.
37. G. Gerig, O. Kübler, R. Kikinis, and F. A. Jolesz. Nonlinear anisotropic filtering of MRI data. *IEEE Transactions on Medical Imaging*, 11:221–232, 1992.
38. S. Ghosal and P. Č. Vaněk. Scalable algorithm for discontinuous optical flow estimation. *IEEE Transactions on Pattern Analysis and Machine Intelligence*, 18(2):181–194, February 1996.
39. F. Glazer. Multilevel relaxation in low-level computer vision. In A. Rosenfeld, editor, *Multiresolution Image Processing and Analysis*, pages 312–330. Springer, Berlin, 1984.
40. W. Hackbusch. *Multigrid Methods and Applications*. Springer, New York, 1985.
41. F. R. Hampel, E. M. Ronchetti, P. J. Rousseeuw, and W. A. Stahel. *Robust Statistics: The Approach Based on Influence Functions*. MIT Press, Cambridge, MA, 1986.
42. F. Heitz and P. Bouthemy. Multimodal estimation of discontinuous optical flow using Markov random fields. *IEEE Transactions on Pattern Analysis and Machine Intelligence*, 15(12):1217–1232, December 1993.
43. W. Hinterberger, O. Scherzer, C. Schnörr, and J. Weickert. Analysis of optical flow models in the framework of calculus of variations. *Numerical Functional Analysis and Optimization*, 23(1/2):69–89, May 2002.
44. B. Horn and B. Schunck. Determining optical flow. *Artificial Intelligence*, 17:185–203, 1981.
45. P. J. Huber. *Robust Statistics*. Wiley, New York, 1981.
46. T. Iijima. Basic theory of pattern observation. In *Papers of Technical Group on Automata and Automatic Control*. IECE, Japan, December 1959. In Japanese.
47. T. Iijima. Observation theory of two-dimensional visual patterns. In *Papers of Technical Group on Automata and Automatic Control*. IECE, Japan, October 1962. In Japanese.
48. S. Ju, M. Black, and A. Jepson. Skin and bones: multi-layer, locally affine, optical flow and regularization with transparency. In *Proc. 1996 IEEE Computer Society Conference on Computer Vision and Pattern Recognition*, pages 307–314, San Francisco, CA, June 1996. IEEE Computer Society Press.
49. J. Karlholm. *Local Signal Models for Image Sequence Analysis*. PhD thesis, Linköping University, Sweden, 1998. Dissertation No. 536.
50. R. Kimmel, R. Malladi, and N. Sochen. Images as embedded maps and minimal surfaces: movies, color, texture, and volumetric medical images. *International Journal of Computer Vision*, 39(2):111–129, September 2000.
51. T. Kohlberger, C. Schnörr, A. Bruhn, and J. Weickert. Parallel variational motion estimation by domain decomposition and cluster computing. In T. Pajdla and J. Matas, editors, *Computer Vision – ECCV 2004, Part IV*, volume 3024 of *Lecture Notes in Computer Science*, pages 205–216. Springer, Berlin, 2004.
52. A. Kumar, A. R. Tannenbaum, and G. J. Balas. Optic flow: a curve evolution approach. *IEEE Transactions on Image Processing*, 5(4):598–610, April 1996.
53. S.-H. Lai and B. C. Vemuri. Reliable and efficient computation of optical flow. *International Journal of Computer Vision*, 29(2):87–105, October 1998.
54. B. Lucas and T. Kanade. An iterative image registration technique with an application to stereo vision. In *Proc. Seventh International Joint Conference on Artificial Intelligence*, pages 674–679, Vancouver, Canada, August 1981.
55. A. Meister. *Numerik linearer Gleichungssysteme*. Vieweg, Braunschweig, 1999.

56. E. Mémin and P. Pérez. Dense estimation and object-based segmentation of the optical flow with robust techniques. *IEEE Transactions on Image Processing*, 7(5):703–719, May 1998.
57. E. Mémin and P. Pérez. A multigrid approach for hierarchical motion estimation. In *Proc. Sixth International Conference on Computer Vision*, pages 933–938, Bombay, India, January 1998. Narosa Publishing House.
58. A. R. Mitchell and D. F. Griffiths. *The Finite Difference Method in Partial Differential Equations*. Wiley, Chichester, 1980.
59. K. W. Morton and L. M. Mayers. *Numerical Solution of Partial Differential Equations*. Cambridge University Press, Cambridge, UK, 1994.
60. H.-H. Nagel. Constraints for the estimation of displacement vector fields from image sequences. In *Proc. Eighth International Joint Conference on Artificial Intelligence*, volume 2, pages 945–951, Karlsruhe, West Germany, August 1983.
61. H.-H. Nagel. Extending the 'oriented smoothness constraint' into the temporal domain and the estimation of derivatives of optical flow. In O. Faugeras, editor, *Computer Vision – ECCV '90*, volume 427 of *Lecture Notes in Computer Science*, pages 139–148. Springer, Berlin, 1990.
62. H.-H. Nagel and W. Enkelmann. An investigation of smoothness constraints for the estimation of displacement vector fields from image sequences. *IEEE Transactions on Pattern Analysis and Machine Intelligence*, 8:565–593, 1986.
63. H.-H. Nagel and A. Gehrke. Spatiotemporally adaptive estimation and segmentation of OF-fields. In H. Burkhardt and B. Neumann, editors, *Computer Vision – ECCV '98*, volume 1407 of *Lecture Notes in Computer Science*, pages 86–102. Springer, Berlin, 1998.
64. M. Z. Nashed and O. Scherzer. Least squares and bounded variation regularization with nondifferentiable functionals. *Numerical Functional Analysis and Optimization*, 19:873–901, 1998.
65. P. Nesi. Variational approach to optical flow estimation managing discontinuities. *Image and Vision Computing*, 11(7):419–439, September 1993.
66. E. P. Ong and M. Spann. Robust optical flow computation based on least-median-of-squares regression. *International Journal of Computer Vision*, 31(1):51–82, 1999.
67. W. H. Press, S. A. Teukolsky, W. T. Vetterling, and B. P. Flannery. *Numerical Recipes in C*. Cambridge University Press, Cambridge, UK, second edition, 1992.
68. M. Proesmans, L. Van Gool, E. Pauwels, and A. Oosterlinck. Determination of optical flow and its discontinuities using non-linear diffusion. In J.-O. Eklundh, editor, *Computer Vision – ECCV '94*, volume 801 of *Lecture Notes in Computer Science*, pages 295–304. Springer, Berlin, 1994.
69. A. R. Rao and B. G. Schunck. Computing oriented texture fields. *CVGIP: Graphical Models and Image Processing*, 53:157–185, 1991.
70. L. I. Rudin, S. Osher, and E. Fatemi. Nonlinear total variation based noise removal algorithms. *Physica D*, 60:259–268, 1992.
71. Y. Saad. *Iterative Methods for Sparse Linear Systems*. SIAM, Philadelphia, second edition, 2003.
72. G. Sapiro. *Geometric Partial Differential Equations and Image Analysis*. Cambridge University Press, Cambridge, UK, 2001.
73. C. Schnörr. Segmentation of visual motion by minimizing convex non-quadratic functionals. In *Proc. Twelfth International Conference on Pattern Recognition*, volume A, pages 661–663, Jerusalem, Israel, October 1994. IEEE Computer Society Press.

74. C. Schnörr. Unique reconstruction of piecewise smooth images by minimizing strictly convex non-quadratic functionals. *Journal of Mathematical Imaging and Vision*, 4:189–198, 1994.
75. C. Schnörr. Convex variational segmentation of multi-channel images. In M.-O. Berger, R. Deriche, I. Herlin, J. Jaffré, and J.-M. Morel, editors, *ICAOS '96: Images, Wavelets and PDEs*, volume 219 of *Lecture Notes in Control and Information Sciences*, pages 201–207. Springer, London, 1996.
76. G. D. Smith. *Numerical Solution of Partial Differential Equations: Finite Difference Methods*. Clarendon Press, Oxford, third edition, 1985.
77. R. Szeliski and J. Coughlan. Hierarchical spline-based image registration. In *Proc. 1994 IEEE Computer Society Conference on Computer Vision and Pattern Recognition*, pages 194–201, Seattle, WA, June 1994. IEEE Computer Society Press.
78. D. Terzopoulos. Image analysis using multigrid relaxation. *IEEE Transactions on Pattern Analysis and Machine Intelligence*, 8(2):129–139, March 1986.
79. A. N. Tikhonov. Solution of incorrectly formulated problems and the regularization method. *Soviet Mathematics Doklady*, 4:1035–1038, 1963.
80. U. Trottenberg, C. Oosterlee, and A. Schüller. *Multigrid*. Academic Press, San Diego, 2001.
81. D. Tschumperlé and R. Deriche. Diffusion tensor regularization with constraints preservation. In *Proc. 2001 IEEE Computer Society Conference on Computer Vision and Pattern Recognition*, volume 1, pages 948–953, Kauai, HI, December 2001. IEEE Computer Society Press.
82. D. Tschumperlé and R. Deriche. Diffusion PDE's on vector-valued images. *IEEE Signal Processing Magazine*, 19(5):16–25, 2002.
83. S. Uras, F. Girosi, A. Verri, and V. Torre. A computational approach to motion perception. *Biological Cybernetics*, 60:79–87, 1988.
84. R. A. Varga. *Matrix Iterative Analysis*. Springer, New York, second edition, 2000.
85. R. Wait and A. R. Mitchell. *Finite Element Analysis and Applications*. Wiley, Chichester, 1985.
86. J. Weber and J. Malik. Robust computation of optical flow in a multi-scale differential framework. *International Journal of Computer Vision*, 14:67–81, 1995.
87. J. Weickert. Scale-space properties of nonlinear diffusion filtering with a diffusion tensor. Technical Report 110, Laboratory of Technomathematics, University of Kaiserslautern, Germany, October 1994.
88. J. Weickert. Coherence-enhancing diffusion of colour images. *Image and Vision Computing*, 17(3–4):199–210, March 1999.
89. J. Weickert and T. Brox. Diffusion and regularization of vector- and matrix-valued images. In M. Z. Nashed and O. Scherzer, editors, *Inverse Problems, Image Analysis, and Medical Imaging*, volume 313 of *Contemporary Mathematics*, pages 251–268. AMS, Providence, 2002.
90. J. Weickert, A. Bruhn, N. Papenberg, and T. Brox. Variational optic flow computation: From continuous models to algorithms. In L. Alvarez, editor, *IWCVIA '03: International Workshop on Computer Vision and Image Analysis*, volume 0026 of *Cuardernos del Instituto Universitario de Ciencias y Technologías Cibernéticas*, pages 1–6, Spain, February 2004.
91. J. Weickert and C. Schnörr. A theoretical framework for convex regularizers in PDE-based computation of image motion. *International Journal of Computer Vision*, 45(3):245–264, December 2001.

92. J. Weickert and C. Schnörr. Variational optic flow computation with a spatio-temporal smoothness constraint. *Journal of Mathematical Imaging and Vision*, 14(3):245–255, May 2001.
93. P. Wesseling. *An Introduction to Multigrid Methods*. R. T. Edwards, Flourtown, 2004.
94. D. M. Young. *Iterative Solution of Large Linear Systems*. Dover, New York, 2003.
95. G. Zini, A. Sarti, and C. Lamberti. Application of continuum theory and multi-grid methods to motion evaluation from 3D echocardiography. *IEEE Transactions on Ultrasonics, Ferroelectrics, and Frequency Control*, 44(2):297–308, March 1997.

Part II

Applications

Fast Image Matching for Generation of Panorama Ultrasound

Armin Schoisswohl

GE Medical Systems Kretz Ultrasound, Austria `armin.schoisswohl@med.ge.com`

Summary Panorama imaging is a key technology for enlarging the view in medical diagnostic ultrasound. Due to the high acquisition data rate and the relatively noisy image data it is a challenging task to performe panorama imaging with software implementation in real-time. A multiscale approach for image matching is presented which meets the requirements in terms of runtime performance and stability.

Keywords medical ultrasound imaging, panorama images, image matching, registration, multilevel optimization

1 Introduction

Medical ultrasound imaging is widely used in various medical applications like Cardiology, Radiology, Obstetrics and Gynecology. Besides of having no negative effects on the human body, its main advantage is that examination results are obtained in real-time providing immediate feedback to the operator.

Ultrasound images are obtained by sending focussed mechanical oszillations of several MHz into the human body and receiving the echoes generated by the scatterers inside the tissue. The ultrasound transducer consists of a 1D array of piezoelectric elements which are excited in a time-delayed manner to form a spheriacal, focussed wave. This same concept of beamforming is used on receive, where the signal is formed by a delay-and-sum approach. The aperture of the array antenna is usually limited by the number of system channels and the size of the elements, which is in the range of half wavelength in order to get sufficient image quality. A thorough introduction to ultrasonic beamforming is given by Anderson and Trahey [17].

As a result of the limited aperture only a limited view can be obtained with a fixed transducer position. However, in many applications it is desirable to get a more comprehensive overview of the region of investigation. This problem can be overcome by recovering in-plane transducer motions and combining the information into a single compound image (Figure 1).

The problem of computing the motion between images is referred to as registration and can be classified into several groups [15, 16]:

- Feature based methods [6, 7] compute the displacement of a small number of characteristic features, so-called landmarks. In general these have to be assigned manually, which is a time-intensive and sometimes quite difficult task.

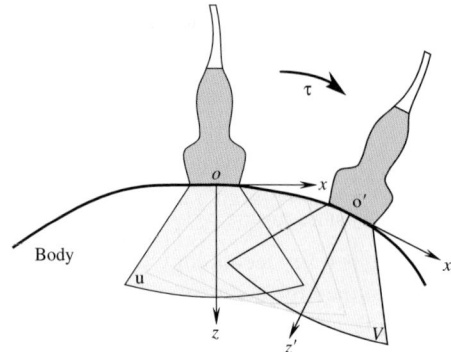

Fig. 1. Principle of creating an extended view: The probe is moved in-plane during the acquisition; in order to overlay the images to form a compound panorama image the geometric transform τ, which describes the probe movement has to be recovered.

- Especially in ultrasound imaging compound images are often generated using external position sensing systems to receive the exact spatial displacement of the image data [14, 13]. This in particular requires additional hardware.
- Image matching methods are based on the optimization of a similarity measure between images and typically work without user interaction. A typical example of such a similarity measure is mutual information which is used for matching images of different modalities (e.g., CT and MRI data [12]). For matching of data which were acquired with the same imaging system often L^2-measures are considered [5, 8]. Excellent sources for additional information on this topic are [11, 9].

Methods for extended ultrasound imaging based on image matching methods have been presented in [19, 20, 18]. There the authors suggest to find translations of sub-image regions and to recover a full isometric affine transformation (rotation and translation) from the individual sub-translations. These algorithms have been released to the market in 1996 under the trademark SieScape^{TM} by Siemens Ultrasound. For image data acquired with small rotations these algorithms have proven to be reliable and stable.

The focus of this article is on the computation of the full in-plane transducer motion that can be described by a rotation and a translation in a fast and reliable way.

2 Problem Formulation

In the following we will consider the recovery of the transformation between two successive images u and v of an image sequence. We assume real valued images defined on a subset Ω of the spatial domain $\mathbb{R}^2$:

$$u : \Omega \subset \mathbb{R}^2 \to \mathbb{R}.$$

The idea of image matching is to find a suitable spatial transformation $\tau : \mathbb{R}^2 \to \mathbb{R}^2$ such that the two successive images u and v are similar on their intersectioning domain, i.e.,

$$u(\tau(x)) = v(x). \tag{1}$$

In reality there may not exist a solution of (1) due to noise and different acquisition conditions (like deformations, illumination changes, etc). Therefore, instead of looking for a solution of (1), we aim to minimize a similarity measure between $u(\tau)$ and v in a suitable class of transformations $\mathcal{T}$.

3 A Constrained Optimization Problem

The application of image matching considered in this paper is the generation of panorama images, i.e., different views of a single static object have to be compounded. The model for the admissible movements here is exactly all in-plane translations and rotations of the transducer; there it makes sense to restrict the admissible mappings to the set of isometric affine transformations, which are exactly compositions of a rotation and a translation, i.e.,

$$\mathcal{T} := \{\tau = \tau(\varphi, b) : \mathbb{R}^2 \to \mathbb{R}^2, x \mapsto R(\varphi)x + b\}.$$

This in particular means that all admissible mappings $\tau \in \mathcal{T}$ can be parameterized by the tuple (φ, b), with the rotation angle $\varphi \in (-\pi, \pi)$ and the translation vector $b \in \mathbb{R}^2$.

The similarity of the remapped image $u(\tau)$ and v can be measured by the L^2-error

$$\varepsilon(\tau) := \int (u(\tau(x)) - v(x))^2 \, dx.$$

If both images contain the whole object surrounded by an identical background (e.g., horizontal CT slices), then the dependency of the functional ε from the overlapping domain $\Omega(\tau)$ can be eliminated by extending the data sets in an appropriate way. Matching problems of this kind are tackled by solving the Euler equations [5, 8].

However, as already mentioned in the introduction, Ultrasound data is given on a finite domain $\Omega \subset \mathbb{R}^2$. Thus, after transformation the displaced image $u(\tau)$ is defined on the set $\tau^{-1}(\Omega)$ which, in general, is different from Ω, and there is no information available on how to extend the image beyond its boundaries. Therefore the intersection of the two images has to be taken into account. This can be done with the relative L^2-error functional of [3]

$$\frac{\int_{\Omega(\tau)} (u(\tau(x)) - v(x))^2 dx}{|\Omega(\tau)|}$$

in the domain of overlap $\Omega(\tau)$ of the images u and v

$$\Omega(\tau) := \tau^{-1}(\Omega) \cap \Omega.$$

However, we propose to address the intersection problem by considering the modified L^2 error functional

$$\varepsilon_{u,v}(\tau) := \frac{\int_{\mathbb{R}^2} \chi\bigl(u(\tau(x))\bigr) \cdot \chi\bigl(v(x)\bigr) \cdot \bigl(u(\tau(x)) - v(x)\bigr)^2 dx}{\int_{\mathbb{R}^2} \chi\bigl(u(\tau(x))\bigr) \cdot \chi\bigl(v(x)\bigr) dx}, \qquad (2)$$

where χ is an appropriately chosen function. We suppose that

$$u(x) = v(x) := 0 \qquad \text{for all } x \notin \Omega.$$

The particular choice of the function $\chi : \mathbb{R} \to \mathbb{R}$ can be used to suppress or emphasize certain image intensities, e.g., neglect differences if one image is below some threshold. In practice it turned out that setting χ to the identity function $\chi(s) = s$ is a reasonable choice.

The problem of finding the matching transformation τ_k between the two successive image u_k and u_{k+1} of an image sequence can now be written as finding the minimizer of the functional $\varepsilon_{u,v}$ from (2), i.e.,

$$\tau_{u,v} := \arg\min_{\tau \in \mathcal{T}} \varepsilon_{u,v}(\tau),$$

4 Multiscale Optimization

In practical implementation the functional ε from (2) shows many local extrema that are caused by image features, and are also due to the interpolation that has to be used when evaluating the image transformations (Figure 2).

In order to stabilize and speedup the optimization procedure, we propose a multiresolution approach for minimizing ε over $\mathcal{T}$:

1. For two images u and v we compute a series of approximations

$$u_m := P_m u, \quad v_m := P_m v, \quad (m = 0, \ldots, M)$$

of decreasing resolution m; here P_m denotes the projection onto the space V_m, where $\{V_m\}$ is a series of approximation spaces of decreasing resolution. As suggested in [1] we use approximations according to a Laplacian pyramid.

2. Now we use an iterative multilevel technique with respect to the scaling parameter m:
    a) We specify the coarsest level $m := M$ and an appropriate initial guess τ^0 — typically the identity mapping.
    b) To minimize the functional

$$\varepsilon_m(\tau) := \varepsilon_{u_m, v_m}(\tau)$$

we use an iterative optimization method with initial guess τ_m^0; here the subscripts indicate the dependency on the input data u_m and v_m.

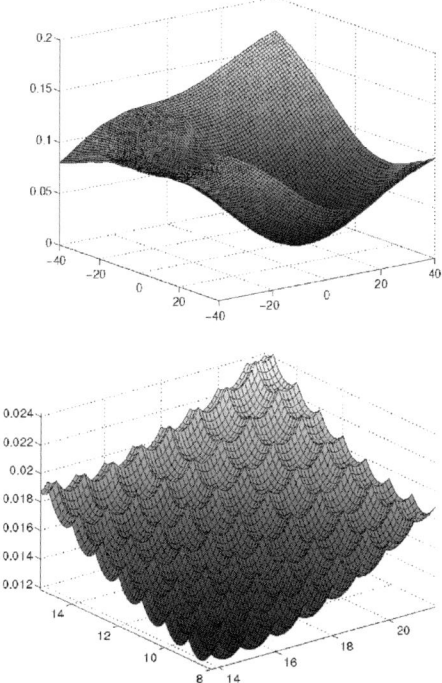

Fig. 2. Plot of the error functional $\varepsilon(\tau)$ for 2D input data; displacements are restricted to translations $\tau = \tau(0, b)$: the zoom (bottom) shows the ripples introduced by image interpolation.

c) The minimizer $\tau_m = (\varphi_m, b_m)$ of the functional ε_m is used as initial guess τ_{m-1}^0 at the next finer level $m := m - 1$ and we proceed with step 2b until $m = 0$ or an appropriate stopping criterion is satisfied.

This approach has two advantages: first, the functional ε_m is smoother than ε and has less local minima. Moreover the computational effort for evaluating ε_m is significantly smaller compared to the effort for evaluating ε since the projected data sets u_m, v_m are significantly smaller (by a factor of 4^m). Once an approximation τ_m has been obtained the optimization algorithm on the next finer scale $m - 1$ requires only a few iterations due to a good initial guess τ_{m-1}^0.

In comparison with ε the functional ε_m has significantly less local minima. However the ripples caused by interpolation are still significant. Experiments showed that optimization methods utilizing derivatives (like e.g., the Levenberg–Marquardt method as suggested in [3, 1]) are sometimes too sensitive to the local minima introduced by the ripples.

We therefore propose to use the Hooke–Jeeves optimization algorithm [2], a direct search method that has been designed specifically for the optimization of non-smooth functionals. This method does not perform any line search but rather takes discrete steps along search directions (usually the coordinate directions of the parameter space), where the size of the steps is decreased during the optimization procedure, thus avoiding to be trapped into small local minima. A good overview about this method is given in [4].

5 Numerical Results

This section presents some results that show the performance and stability of the proposed method for image matching. For measuring the accuracy of the method we used the synthetic image data as shown in Figure 3: a blurred bright square on dark background of 512 by 512 pixels. For experiments using noisy data we distorted this image by Gaussian white noise of 10dB PSNR which had been smoothed by a Gaussian window to resemble more closely the appearance of ultrasound data.

The proposed algorithm has been implemented in C on a Intel Pentium 4 processor running at 2 GHz. The code makes use of Intel's Performance Primitives [21], a collection of highly processor specific optimized image and signal processing routines. CPU times were measured from the CPU's cycle counter meaning that the processing times include some overhead originating from the operating system.

5.1 Experiments using Synthetic Data

In a first test we shifted the undisturbed image by an amount of 13.7 pixels horizontally and 7.4 pixels vertically. This image was matched with the original image. Figure 4 shows the progress of the multi-scale Hooke-Jeeves optimization. It is clearly visible that the optimal solution is approached rapidly at the coarse approximation level (upper two rows), where iterations are computationally inexpensive due to the small amount of data of the approximations from the Laplacian pyramid. It can also be noticed that the Hooke-Jeeves iterations themselves show good performance when approaching the optimum in big steps at the beginning and refining the solution in finer steps subsequently.

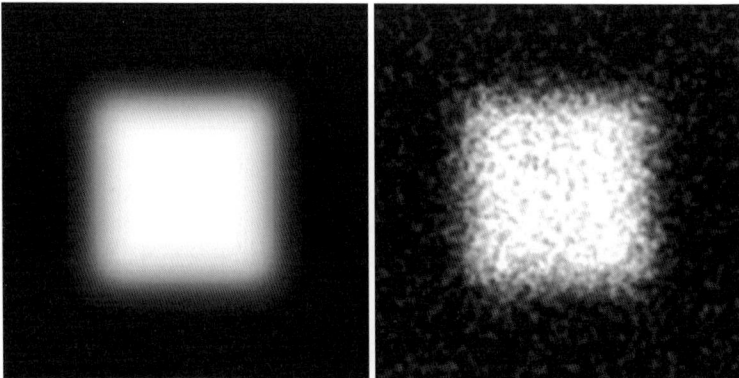

Fig. 3. Sythetic test datasets without noise (left) and with noise of 10dB PSNR (right)

Fast Image Matching for Generation of Panorama Ultrasound 145

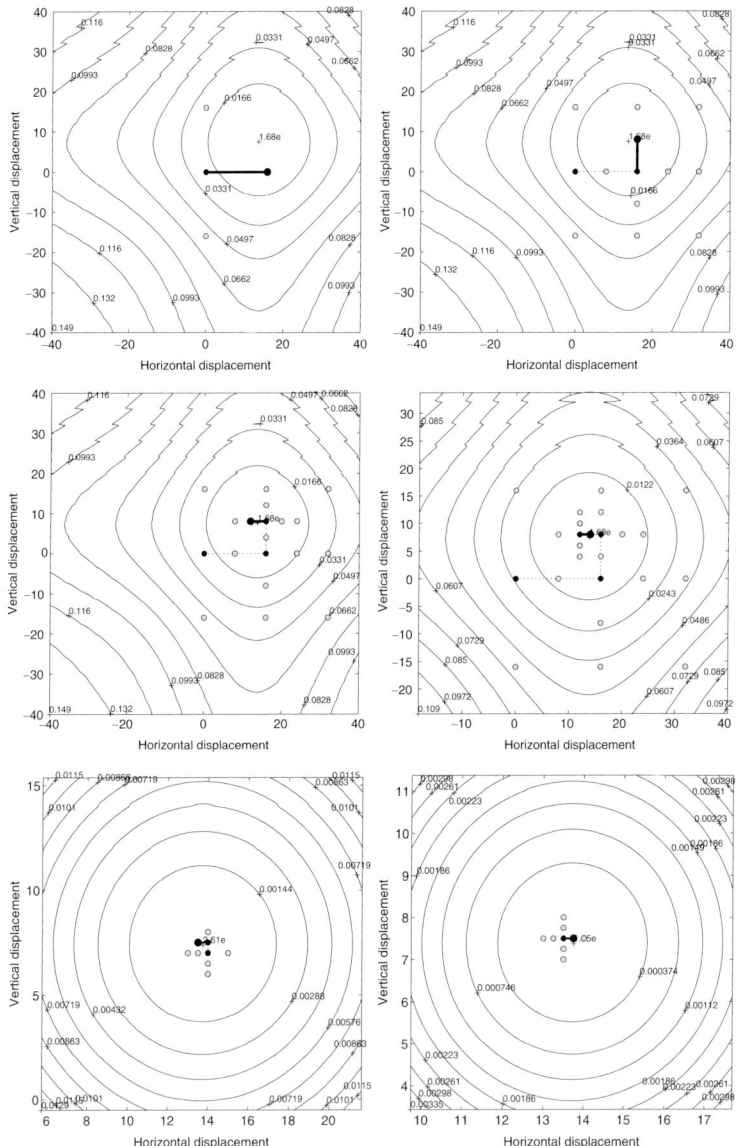

Fig. 4. Progress of optimization on test data set from Figure 3: Black spots denote base points of the Hooke-Jeeves Algorithm, circles denote explored points. Intermediate results are shown for translation only for image scale 4 (upper two rows) and the results for scale 3 and 2 (bottom row)

On the finer levels from the Laplacian pyramid the result is refined only marginally. Therefore only few iterations have to be carried out.

Figure 5 shows the progess of the optimization over computing time - both the value of the error functional as well as the relative error plotted versus CPU time. These graphs again show that the optimum is approached rapidly on the coarse scales, where iterations are relatively inexpensive. At finer levels only a few iterations are needed.

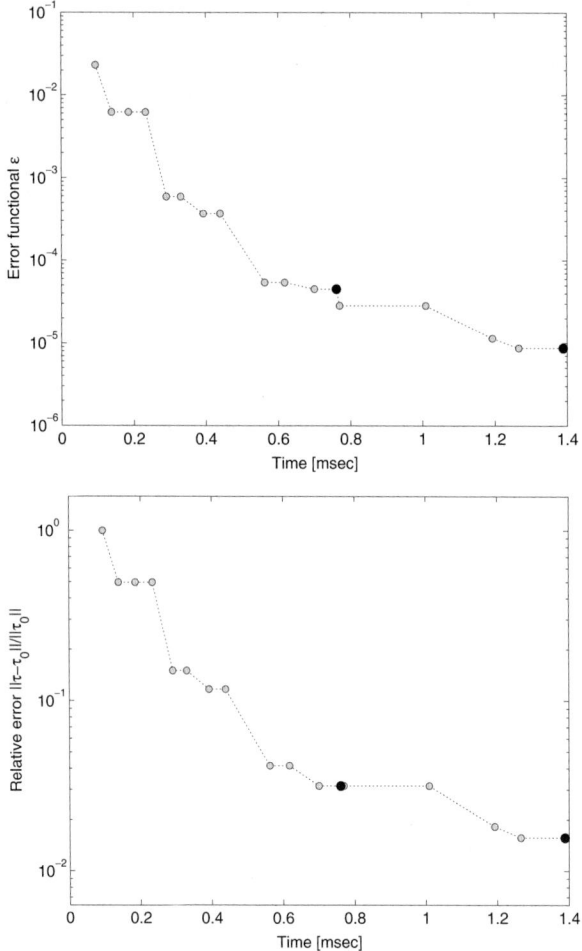

Fig. 5. Progress of optimization on test data set from Figure 3: functional value versus CPU-time (top) and relative error of parameter guess versus CPU-time (bottom). Dark spots denote the solution on a specific image scale.

5.2 Experiments using Noisy Data

The experiments from the previous section were repeated using noisy data (Figure 3, right). The results are basically identical to the results using non-distorted data: The optimum is approached fast on the coarse levels, and subsequently on finer levels only a few iterations are needed. The results are shown in Figures 6 and 7.

5.3 Multi-scale Hooke-Jeeves Performance

We also compared the performance of the usual Hooke-Jeeves optimization and the multi-scale Hooke-Jeeves optimization as proposed in this article. Figure 8 shows that the multi-scale approach reduces the CPU time by more than 50% (3.1sec vs. 6.8sec). Although this improvement by a multi-scale aproach is not as significant as found in combination with other optimization techniques [3], it is still significant enough, especially when dealing with real time performance requirements: 3.1 CPU seconds means that about 30 frames per second can be processed.

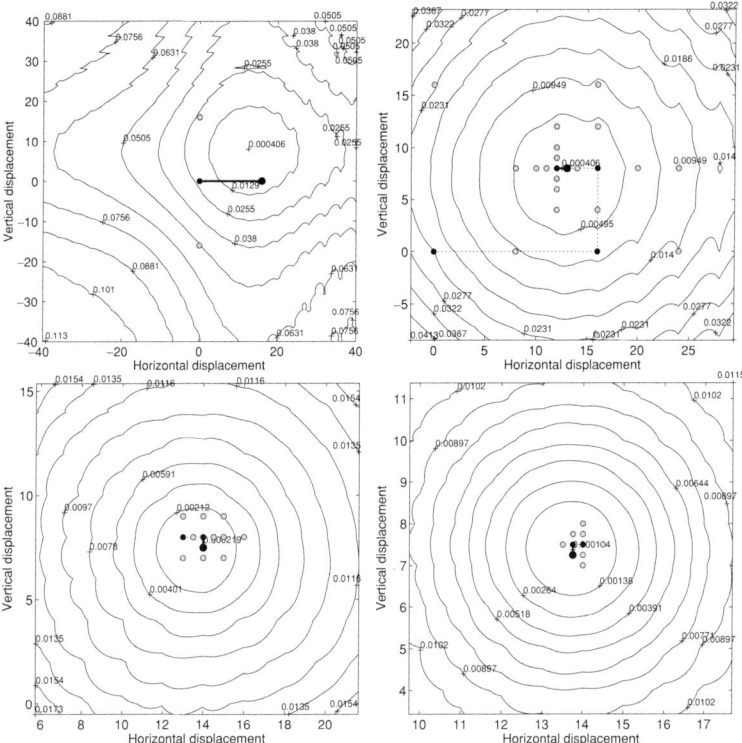

Fig. 6. Progress of optimization on noisy test data set from Figure 3: Black spots denote base points of the Hooke-Jeeves Algorithm, circles denote explored points. Start on level 4 (top left), results on level 4 (top right), level 3 (bottom left) and level 2 (bottom right)

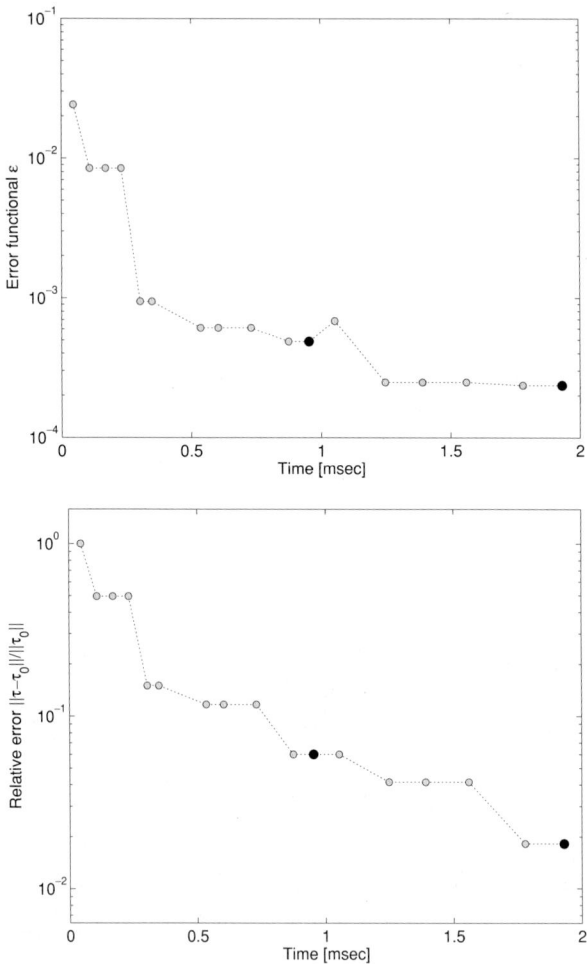

Fig. 7. Progress of optimization on noisy test data set from Figure 3: functional value versus CPU-time (top) and relative error of parameter guess versus CPU-time (bottom). Dark spots denote the solution on a specific image scale.

Finally in Figure 9 we show a result as shown in the implementation of the proposed method on a commercial Ultrasound scanner. The panorama image has been generated from 3 second sweeps at an acquisition frame rate of 44Hz, i.e., from about 130 images. For displaying the displaced images have been combined using averaging techniques.

Fast Image Matching for Generation of Panorama Ultrasound   149

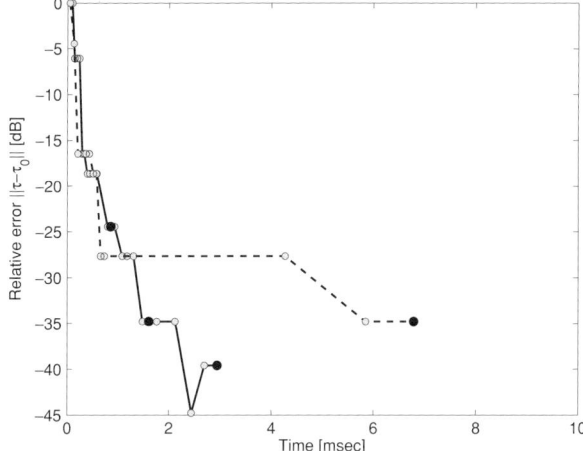

Fig. 8. Progress of optimization on noisy test data set from Figure 3: relative error of parameter guess versus CPU-time. The multiscale approach (solid) shows an additional speedup compared to the single scale approach (dashed).

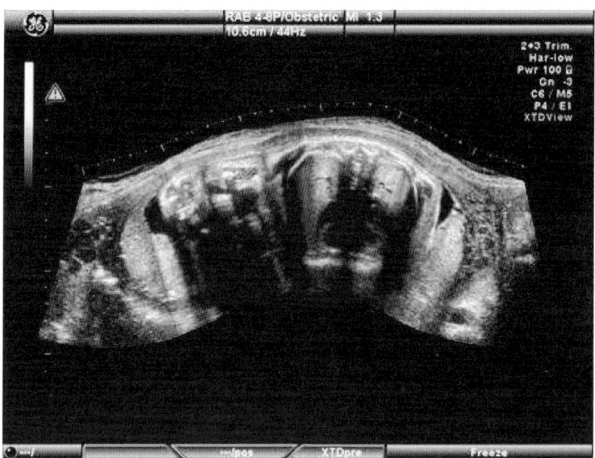

Fig. 9. Result as shown in the implementation on a commercial Ultrasound Scanner. The image is generated from a 3 second sweep acquired at a framerate of 44Hz

References

1. P. Thévenaz, U. E. Ruttimann and M. Unser: A Pyramid Approach to Subpixel Registration Based on Intensity. IEEE Transactions on Image Processing, **7/1**, pp 27-41 (1998)
2. R. Hooke and T.A. Jeeves: "Direct search" solution of numerical and statistical problems, JACM **8/2**, pp 212-229 (1961)
3. O. Scherzer and A. Schoisswohl: A fast and robust algorithm for 2D/3D panorama ultrasound data, Real-Time Imaging **8/1**, pp 53-60 (2002)

4. C. T. Kelley: Iterative methods for optimization, SIAM Frontiers in applied mathematics, Philadelphia **18**, (1999)
5. Y. Amit: A nonlinear variational problem for image matching, SIAM J. Sci. Comput **15/1**, pp 207-224 (1994)
6. R. Boesecke, T. Bruckner and G. Ende: Landmark based correlation of medical images, Phys. Med. Biol **35**, pp 121-129 (1990)
7. F. L. Bookstein: Size and shape spaces for landmark data in two dimensions, Statist. Sci. **1**, pp 181-242 (1986)
8. B. Fischer and J. Modersitzky: Fast inversion of matrices arising in image processing, Num. Alg. **22**, pp 1-11 (1999)
9. T. McInerney and D. Terzopoulos: Deformable models in medical image analysis: a survey, Medical Image Analysis **1/2**, pp 91-108 (1996)
10. G. P. Penney, J. Weese, A. J. Little, P. Desmedt, D. L. G. Hill and D. J. Hawkes: A comparison of similarity measures for use in 2D-3D medical image registration, IEEE Trans. Med. Imag. **17**, pp 586-595 (1998)
11. D.L.G. Hill: Combination of 3D medical images from multiple modalities. PhD Thesis, University of London (1993)
12. C. Studholme, D. L. G. Hill and D. J. Hawkes: Automated 3D registration of MR and CT images of the head. Medical Image Analysis **1/2**, pp 163–175 (1996)
13. R. Rohling, A Gee and L. Berman: Three-dimensional spatial compounding of ultrasound images. Medical Image Analysis **1/3**, pp 177–193 (1996)
14. H. Erbe, A. Kriete, A Jödicke, W. Deinsberger and D. K. Böker: 3D-Ultrasonography and image matching for detection of brain shift during intracranial surgery. CAR'96 Computer Assisted Radiology by Lemke, H.U. and Vannier, M.W. and Inamura, K. and Farman, A.G., International Congress Series, Elsevier Science B.V. **1124**, pp 225–230 (1996)
15. P. Gerlot-Chiron and Y. Bizais: Registration of multimodality medical images using a region overlap criterion, CVGIP: Graphical Models and Images Processing **54/5**, pp 396–406 (1992)
16. P. A. Van den Elsen, E.J.D. Pol, and M. A. Viergever: Medical image matching - a review with classification, IEEE Eng. Med. Biol. Mag **12**, pp 26–39 (1993)
17. M. E. Anderson and G. E. Trahey: A seminar on k-space applied to medical ultrasound, Departement of Biomedical Engineering, Duke University, April (2000)
18. A. Tirumalai, C. Lowery, D. Gustafson and P. Sutcliffe and P. VonBehren: Display and PACS, Extended-Field-of-View Ultrasound Imaging, SPIE, Handbook of Medical Imaging **3**, pp 277-303 (2000)
19. L. Weng and A. P. Tirumalai: Method and apparatus for generating large compound ultrasound image, U.S. Patent No. 5,782,766, Nov (1996)
20. L. Nock, L. Weng and A. P. Tirumalai: Method and apparatus for generating and displaying panoramic ultrasound images, U.S. Patent No. 5,782,766, July (1998)
21. Intel Corp.: Integrated Performance Primitives for Signal and Image Processing, http://developer.intel.com, Version 4.0 (2004)

Inpainting of Movies Using Optical Flow

Harald Grossauer

University of Innsbruck, Institute of Computer Sciences
harald.grossauer@uibk.ac.at

Abstract We consider fully automatic restauration of movie sequences which are distorted by blotches and scratches. Two different approaches are combined:

Firstly, distortions localized within a single frame are detected by analyzing temporal correlations between frames. For this means motion estimation between frames is performed by employing an optical flow computation. An efficient algorithm for the calculation of the optical flow field is described. Regions where the motion estimation gives bad results are considered as distorted. Blotches are repaired by copying appropriate image data from neighboring frames, according to the flow field.

Secondly, distortions extending over several contiguous frames usually appear as narrow, vertical scratches. Since they occur at nearly the same locations in subsequent frames they are not detected by the optical flow. Due to their shape they are easily identified as peaks in the mean column intensity. Mostly image information destroyed by scratches is neither available in adjacent frames. Thus a still image inpainting algorithm is used to reconstruct the lost image contents solely from the available information within one frame.

1 Introduction

A lot of research has been done recently in the area of image inpainting algorithms. The task of this research is to fill in missing (or otherwise destroyed or unwanted) regions in images. The two main approaches thereby considered are with partial differential equations (PDEs), resp., variational based algorithms [1, 2, 3, 4, 5, 6, 7, 8, 9, 10, 11], and texture synthesis algorithms, usually with Markov Random Fields [12, 13, 14, 15, 16, 17]. Some hybrid algorithms have been proposed combining both approaches [18, 19, 20, 21]. There also exist a few algorithms based on different approaches [22, 23, 24, 25]. Most of these algorithms require as input the corrupted image along with a mask highlighting the corrupted regions. This mask has to be created manually by the user. The time needed to create the mask and the computation time of the algorithm usually exceed by far the time needed to perform manual inpainting with standard image processing packages like, e.g., Adobe Photoshop or The GIMP. Besides, the quality of manual inpainting is mostly superior to the results of inpainting algorithms.

The situation is different if a sequence of consecutive images should be restaurated, e.g., restauration of a digitized celluloid movie. Even short movies consist of several thousands of frames with disturbances appearing in random locations in every frame. Thus it is not feasible to manually mark distorted regions. Since consecutive frames differ only marginally and in a mostly predictable way it is possible to detect defects like scratches automatically. Moreover, if a corresponding undisturbed region is found in neighboring frames the image information can be copied from there, thereby omitting still image inpainting algorithms.

Several movie restoration algorithms making use of temporal correlations between frames have already been proposed. One possible approach is to perform spatio-temporal texture synthesis to create dynamic textures, see e.g., [26, 27, 28]. Thereby texture synthesis is performed in three dimensions where adaptions are made to account for the special role of the time dimension. A movie inpainting algorithm employing this approach was presented in [29]. For the examples given in the paper and on the website (short sequences with low resolution) the author reports computation times of two days on average with an unoptimised code.[1] The topic of movie inpainting in general is treated in detail in the extensive work of Kokaram (cf. [30] and the numerous citations therein). The algorithm presented in the current paper relies on similar ideas as in Kokaram's work but while he employs statistical methods we use PDE based techniques. Further Kokaram performs motion estimation block-wise whereas we calculate motion vectors on a per-pixel basis. Like Kokaram we emphasize the importance of coupling the detection and the restauration phase.

The remainder of this paper is built up as follows: in section 2 we introduce the optical flow which is our method for identifying corresponding regions in contiguous frames. In section 3 we introduce a method to detect scratches from the optical flow field. In section 4 we finally present a method for inpainting of frames which makes use of appropriate information in adjacent frames.

2 Optical Flow

The problem of identifying correspondences between frames has a long tradition in computer vision. One of the first approaches was given by Horn & Schunck [31]. Its underlying assumption is that the grey value of an object does not change along its trajectory, i.e.,

$$I(x(t_1), y(t_1); t_1) = I(x(t_2), y(t_2); t_2), \quad \forall t_1, t_2 \qquad (1)$$

or its linearized version

$$\frac{dI(x, y; t)}{dt} = \frac{\partial I}{\partial x} \cdot \frac{dx}{dt} + \frac{\partial I}{\partial y} \cdot \frac{dy}{dt} + \frac{\partial I}{\partial t} = 0 \qquad (2)$$

where $(x(t), y(t))$ denotes the "trajectory" of a pixel. (1) is called the *grey value constancy condition* (GVC condition), (2) is the famous *optical flow constraint*. By introducing the *optical flow field* $\mathbf{h}(t) := (u(t), v(t)) := \left(\frac{dx}{dt}, \frac{dy}{dt}\right)$ (2) can also be written as

---
[1] Private communication with the author

$$\frac{\partial I}{\partial t} = -\nabla I \cdot \mathbf{h}. \tag{3}$$

Two issues are important. Firstly, (2) is one equation for two unknown functions (u, v). Secondly, (3) only allows to detect the motion component parallel to the image gradient (the so called *aperture problem*). This problem is common to all image gradient based approaches. The first problem can be overcome by supplementing an additional constraint on the flow field, e.g., smoothness or piecewise smoothness constraints. Several different constraints have been investigated by Nagel & Enkelmann [32].

We make use of a variational formulation for the optical flow problem which is similar to that presented by Brox et.al. [33]. Given two consecutive frames I_1, I_2 : $\Omega \subset \mathbb{R}^2 \to \mathbb{R}$ we search for a displacement field $\mathbf{h} = (u, v)$ that minimizes

$$E(\mathbf{h}) = \int_\Omega \left(\frac{1}{2} (I_1(\mathbf{x}) - I_2(\mathbf{x} + \mathbf{h}))^2 + \alpha \|\nabla \mathbf{h}\| \right) dx. \tag{4}$$

Here α is a weighting parameter controlling the influence of the *smoothness term* $\|\nabla \mathbf{h}\|$, the Frobenius norm of the Jacobian matrix $\nabla \mathbf{h}$. For an analysis of energy functionals like (4) we confer to [34].

2.1 Optimality Condition and Numerical Implementation

To find a minimizer of functional (4) we employ a gradient descent approach, i.e., we introduce an artificial time parameter and solve the parabolic differential equation

$$\frac{\partial \mathbf{h}}{\partial t} = -E'(\mathbf{h}) \tag{5}$$

up to a stationary point in time. All along this work we assume homogeneous Neumann boundary data for $\mathbf{h}$. Thus

$$-E'(\mathbf{h}) = (I_1(\mathbf{x}) - I_2(\mathbf{x} + \mathbf{h})) \cdot (\nabla I_2)|_{\mathbf{x}+\mathbf{h}} + \alpha \nabla \left(\frac{\nabla \mathbf{h}}{\|\nabla \mathbf{h}\|} \right) \tag{6}$$

is the steepest descent direction for $E(\mathbf{h})$. Here $(\nabla I_2)|_{\mathbf{x}+\mathbf{h}}$ denotes the gradient of I_2, evaluated at $\mathbf{x} + \mathbf{h}$. (5) depicts a system of two equations, we describe its discretization with the first equation, the second equation goes along analogously. Partial derivatives are denoted by subscript indices, e.g., $I_{2,x} := \frac{\partial I_2}{\partial x}$. Further we abbreviate

$$\phi := \frac{1}{\|\nabla \mathbf{h}\|} = \left(\sqrt{u_x^2 + u_y^2 + v_x^2 + v_y^2 + \beta^2} \right)^{-1}$$

where β is a small regularization parameter to prevent divisions by zero. With this notation discretizing (5) in time results in

$$\frac{u^{n+1} - u^n}{\delta t} = (I_1(\mathbf{x}) - I_2(\mathbf{x} + \mathbf{h}^n)) \cdot I_{2,x}(\mathbf{x} + \mathbf{h}^n) \tag{7}$$
$$+ \alpha \nabla \left(\phi^{n+1} \nabla u^{n+1} \right)$$

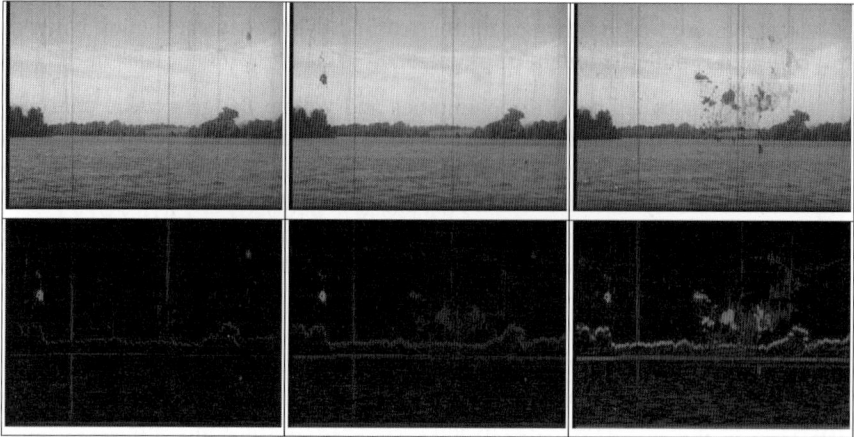

Fig. 1. The upper row shows three consecutive frames of the movie "Flatboatmen of the Frontier", taken from the Prelinger collection on http://www.archive.org. Blotches in the middle picture should be detected. The lower left image shows the difference between the middle frame and the motion compensated left frame, corresponding to $|I_{n-1}(\mathbf{x} + \mathbf{h}_b) - I_n(\mathbf{x})|$. Blotches from both frames appear in the difference image. The lower right image shows the analogous difference for the motion compensated right frame. In the lower middle picture – containing the pixelwise geometric mean of both difference images – only blotches occurring in the middle frame are salient.

3.2 Scratch Detection

Due to mechanical forces in the projector celluloid movies frequently suffer from long vertical scratches spanning several frames. Since they show up at similar positions in neighboring frames they can be matched exactly and thus are not detected by the algorithm described in the previous section. Although there exist several approaches for scratch detection (see [37, 38, 39, 40, 41]) we found the simple algorithm described in the following to be quite successfull. For an image $I: \mathbb{R}^2 \to \mathbb{R}$ let

$$PI(x) = \frac{1}{H} \int_0^H I(x,y) dy \qquad (14)$$

denote its mean intensity at "column" x, where H denotes the height of the image. A scratch is usually a narrow vertical region which is substantially darker (or sometimes brighter) than adjacent columns. Thus scratch locations may be identified as peaks in $PI(x)$, see figure 2. Algorithmically we find scratches as follows: first we calculate $PI(x)$. Since $PI(x)$ has several small extrema we apply a few steps of a one-dimensional bounded variation filter (see, e.g., [42]), which suppresses small extrema but leaves large ones almost undisturbed. Possible peak locations are found as zero-crossings in the first derivative of $PI(x)$ and are accepted as peak if the second derivative is larger than a given threshold, i.e.,

$$(PI)'(x) = 0, \text{ and } |(PI)''(x)| > t. \qquad (15)$$

The width of the scratch is assumed to be twice the distance from the peak to the nearest inflection points at each side (zero-crossings of the second derivative). I.e., if x_p denotes the location of the peak, x_l and x_r denote positions of the nearest inflection points to the left, resp., right of x_p, then the scratch is assumed to cover the interval $[x_p - 2(x_p - x_l), x_p + 2(x_r - x_p)]$.

Obviously this algorithm is very sensitive to narrow, nearly vertical image features, but so are most other scratch detection algorithms. In our test sequences we did not have a single case of a falsely detected scratch.

4 Inpainting of Image Sequences

After distorted locations in the frames have been identified an inpainting algorithm can be applied. Several of them can be found in the reference list. Instead of that, available information can also be transferred from neighboring frames, filling the distorted regions more reliably if corresponding pixels can be found. A natural choice to look for corresponding pixel locations is to use the optical flow fields which have already been computed for the blotch detection. But since for blotches there are usually no matching counterparts in adjacent frames the displacement vectors do not necessarily attain meaningful values. Instead, their values strongly depend on the regularization parameter α, see figure 3. If α is chosen large enough then the regularization term straightens out irregularities in the optical flow field caused by small blotches. Thus the displacement vectors still often point to pixels containing appropriate image information to fill in the blotchy region. Our numerical experiments support this opinion: the results achieved by our algorithm are satisfactory even without post-processing the flow field inside blotch regions.

To fill in missing regions and make use of available data as much as possible we employ the following strategy: in a first step we calculate the forward and backward flow fields for all frames. Using the criteria from section 3.1 blotchy pixels are marked as corrupted. To prevent edge effects the blotch regions are slightly enlarged by performing a morphological dilation. Likewise, by applying the scratch detection from section 3.2, pixels being covered by vertical scratches are identified as corrupted. In the second step we transfer data from frames I_{n-1} and I_{n+1} into I_n. First, image data from I_{n-1} is copied according to the backward flow field $\mathbf{h}_b$, unless $\mathbf{h}_b$ points to a corrupted pixel in I_{n-1}. Second, image data from I_{n+1} is transferred into I_n using the forward flow field $\mathbf{h}_f$, again omitting possibly corrupted pixels in I_{n+1}. In the final third step all remaining corrupted pixels of I_n are treated by the still image inpainting algorithm described in [21, 43].

5 Results

An example for movie inpainting is shown in figure 4. The top left image shows the originally corrupted frame which contains extensive damaged areas. The upper right

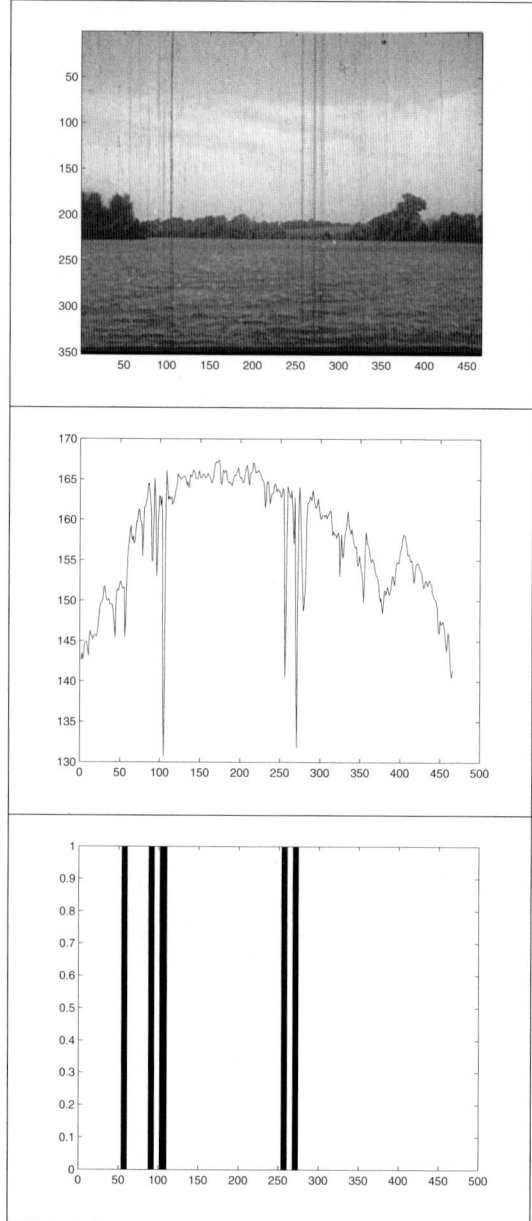

Fig. 2. The uppermost picture shows a frame of the "Flatboatmen"-sequence. The middle picture shows the mean intensity along the columns of the frame. Peaks occur at locations where the frame is scratched. The lower picture indicates all columns which were found by our algorithm to belong to a scratch.

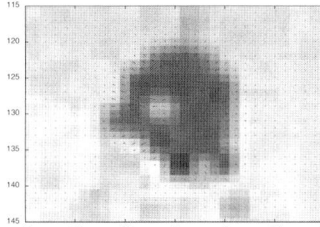 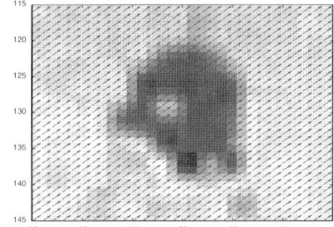

Fig. 3. The influence of the parameter α on the flow field at a blotch. The left image shows the optical flow field with $\alpha = 0.01$, for the right image $\alpha = 0.1$ has been chosen. The length of the arrows is scaled differently for the two images. The "true" motion consists of a panning move towards the lower left.

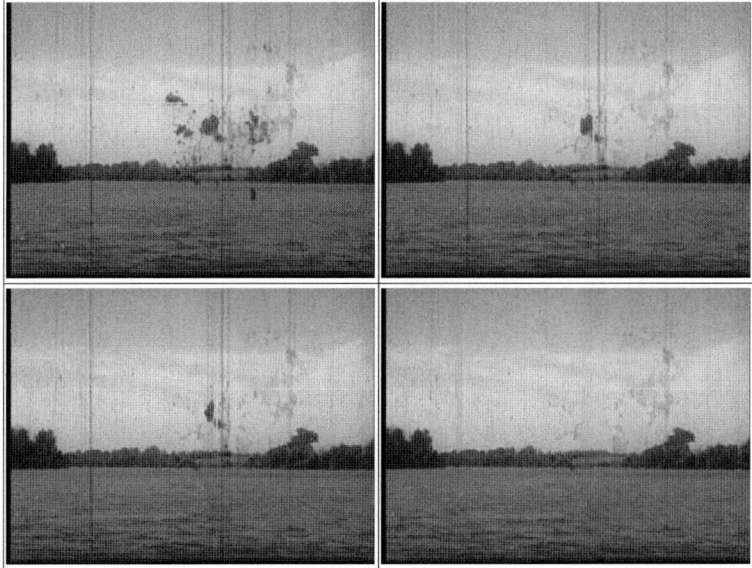

Fig. 4. Progress of movie inpainting. From top left to bottom right: original (corrupted) frame, the same frame after copying corresponding pixels from the previous frame, after copying from the following frame, and after treating remaining corrupted pixels via still image inpainting.

image shows the frame after corresponding pixels have been copied from the previous frame using the backward flow field. A large fraction of the damaged array has already been filled. In the bottom left image additional pixels have been added using the forward flow field and the following frame, which again decreased the size of the blotch. Note that especially the long vertical scratches could not be filled using image information from adjacent frames, since the scratches appear at approximately the same locations. Finally, the bottom right image shows the resulting frame after the still image inpainting algorithm from [21] has been applied.

Acknowledgments

This work was supported by the Austrian Science Fund FWF, grants P15617 and S9207-N12.

References

1. M. Oliveira, B. Bowen, R. McKenna and Y. Chang: Fast Digital Image Inpainting, Proceedings of the International Conference on Visualization, Imaging and Image Processing, (2001)
2. M. Bertalmio, G. Sapiro, V. Caselles and C. Ballester: Image Inpainting, Siggraph 2000, Computer Graphics Proceedings, ACM Press / ACM SIGGRAPH / Addison Wesley Longman, pp 417-424 (2000)
3. M. Bertalmio, A. Bertozzi and G. Sapiro: Navier-Stokes, fluid dynamics, and image and video inpainting, Proc. IEEE Computer Vision and Pattern Recognition (CVPR) (2001)
4. T. Chan and J. Shen: Mathematical Models for Local Nontexture Inpaintings, SIAM Journal on Applied Mathematics, **62/3**, pp 1019–1043, (2002)
5. T. Chan and J. Shen: Non-texture inpaintings by curvature-driven diffusions, J. Visual Comm. Image Rep, **12/4**, pp 436-449, (2001)
6. T. Chan and J. Shen: Morphologically Invariant PDE Inpaintings, Institute for Mathematic and its Applications (IMA), (2001)
7. T. Chan, S. Kang and J. Shen: Euler's elastica and curvature based inpaintings, SIAM J. Applied Mathematics, **63/2**, pp 564-592, (2002)
8. S. Esedoglu and J. Shen: Digital inpainting based on the Mumford-Shah-Euler image model, European J. Appl. Math., (2002)
9. S. Masnou and J. Morel: Level Lines based Disocclusion, Proceedings of ICIP, pp 259-263, (1998)
10. C. Ballester, M. Bertalmio, V. Caselles, G. Sapiro and J. Verdera, Filling-in by joint interpolation of vector fields and grey levels, IEEE Transactions on Image Processing, **10/8**, pp 1200-1211, (2001)
11. H. Grossauer and O. Scherzer: Using the Complex Ginzburg-Landau Equation for Digital Inpainting in 2D and 3D, Scale Space Methods in Computer Vision, LNCS 2695, (2003), pp 225-236
12. H. Igehy and L. Pereira: Image Replacement Through Texture Synthesis, Proceedings of the 1997 IEEE International Conf. on Image Processing, pp 186-189, (1997)
13. P. Harrison: A non-hiearachical procedure for re-synthesis of complex textures, 9-th International Conference in Central Europe on Computer Graphics, Visualization and Computer Vision, pp 190-197, (2001)
14. R.J. Cant and C.S. Langensiepen: A Multiscale Method for Automated Inpainting, 17th European Simulation Multiconference, (2003)
15. I. Drori, D. Cohen-Or and H. Yeshurun: Fragment-based image completion, ACM Transactions on Graphics, **22/3**, pp 303-312, (2003)
16. A. Criminisi, P. Perez and K. Toyama: Object Removal by Exemplar Based Inpainting, Microsoft Research, (2003)
17. J. Jia and C.-K. Tang: Image Repairing: Robust Image Synthesis by Adaptive ND Tensor Voting, IEEE Conference on Computer Vision and Pattern Recognition, pp 643-650, (2003)

18. H. Yamauchi, J. Haber and H.-P. Seidel: Image Restoration using Multiresolution Texture Synthesis and Image Inpainting, Proc. Computer Graphics International, pp 120-125, (2003)
19. M. Bertalmio, L. Vese, G. Sapiro and S. Osher: Simultaneous structure and texture image inpainting, Conference on Computer Vision and Pattern Recognition, **2**, (2003)
20. S. Rane, G. Sapiro and M. Bertalmio: Structure and texture filling-in of missing image blocks in wireless transmission and compression applications, Image Processing, IEEE Transactions, **12/3**, pp 296-303, (2003)
21. H. Grossauer: A Combined PDE and Texture Synthesis Approach to Inpainting, European Conference on Computer Vision, LNCS 3022, (2004), pp 214-224
22. A. Hirani and T. Totsuka: Combining Frequency and Spatial Domain Information for Fast Interactive Image Noise Removal, Computer Graphics, Annual Conference Series, **30**, pp 269-276, (1996)
23. A. Levin, A. Zomet and Y. Weiss: Learning How to Inpaint from Global Image Statistics, Ninth IEEE International Conference on Computer Vision, **1**, pp 305, (2003)
24. V. Savchenko, N. Kojekine and H. Unno: A Practical Image Retouching Method, Proceedings of The First International IEEE Symposium on Cyber Worlds, (2002)
25. S. Rane, J. Remus and G. Sapiro: Wavelet-Domain Reconstruction of Lost Blocks in Wireless Image Transmission and Packet-Switched Networks, IEEE 2002 International Conference on Image Processing, (2002)
26. Z. Bar-Joseph, R. El-Yaniv, D. Lischinski and W. Werman: Texture mixing and texture movie synthesis using statistical learning, IEEE Transactions on Visualization and Computer Graphics, **7/2**, (2001)
27. G. Doretto, E. Jones and S. Soatto: Spatially Homogeneous Dynamic Textures, European Conference on Computer Vision, LNCS 3022, (2004)
28. L. Yuan, F. Wen, C. Liu and H.-Y. Shun: Synthesizing Dynamic Texture with Closed-Loop Linear Dynamic System, European Conference on Computer Vision, LNCS 3022, (2004)
29. Y. Wexler, E. Shechtman and M. Irani: Space-Time Video Completion, Computer Vision and Pattern Recognition (CVPR), (2004)
30. A. Kokaram: Practical, Unified, Motion and Missing Data Treatment in Degraded Video, Journal of Mathematical Imaging and Vision, **20**, (2004)
31. B. K. P. Horn and B. G. Schunck: Determining Optical Flow, Artificial Intelligence, **17**, pp 185-204, (1981)
32. H.-H. Nagel and W. Enkelmann: An Investigation of Smoothness Constraints for the Estimation of Displacement Vector Fields from Image Sequences, IEEE Transactions on Pattern Analysis and Machine Intelligence, **5**, pp 565-593, (1986)
33. T. Brox, A. Bruhn, N. Papenberg and Joachim Weickert: High Accuracy Optical Flow Estimation Based on a Theory for Warping, Proceedings of ECCV, LNCS 3024, pp 25-36, (2004)
34. W. Hinterberger, O. Scherzer, C. Schnörr and J. Weickert: Analysis of optical flow models in the framework of calculus of variations, Numerical Functional Analysis and Optimization, **23/1-2**, pp 69-89, (May 2002)
35. P. Perona and J. Malik: Scale–Space and Edge Detection Using Anisotropic Diffusion, IEEE Trans. on Pattern Analysis and Machine Intelligence, **12/7**, (1990)
36. J. Weickert: Anisotropic diffusion in image processing, European Consortium for Mathematics in Industry, B. G. Teubner, Stuttgart, (1998)
37. M. Nadenau and S. Mitra: Blotch and Scratch Detection in Image Sequences based on Rank Ordered Differences, 5th International Workshop on Time-Varying Image Processing and Moving Object Recognition, Florence, Italy, (1996)

38. S. Godsill and A. Kokaram: Restoration of image sequences using a causal spatio temporal model, The Art and Science of Bayesian Image Analysis, pp 189-194, (1997)
39. L. Joyeux, O. Buisson, B. Besserer and S. Boukir: Detection and removal of line scratches in motion picture films, Proc. CVPR'99, IEEE Int. Conf. on Computer Vision and Pattern Recognition, (1999)
40. B. Besserer and C. Thire: Detection and Tracking Scheme for Line Scratch Removal in an Image Sequence, LNCS 3023, Proceedings of ECCV '04, pp 264-275, (2004)
41. D. Vitulano, V. Bruni and P. Ciarlini: Line Scratch Detection on Digital Images: An Energy Based Model, 10-th International Conference in Central Europe on Computer Graphics, Visualization and Computer Vision, (2002)
42. W. Hinterberger, M. Hintermüller, K. Kunisch, M. Oehsen and O. Scherzer: Tube methods for BV-regularization, Journal of Mathematical Imaging and Vision, **19**, 223-238, (2003)
43. H. Grossauer: Completion of Images with Missing Data Regions, PhD. thesis, Department of Computer Science, University of Innsbruck, Austria

Part III

Medical Applications

Multimodality Registration in Daily Clinical Practice

Reto Bale

Universitätsklinik für Radiodiagnostik, SIP-Labor `reto.bale@uibk.ac.at`

Introduction The discovery of x-rays by Wilhelm Conrad Röntgen in 1895 revolutionized medicine. The novel technology permitted to investigate internal structures of the body without surgery in a non-invasive manner. In the meantime many different imaging modalities have been developed allowing for non-invasive and painless examination of the patient. In contrast to plain x-ray images modern tomographic imaging technologies allow to reconstruct cross-sectional images providing superposition-free images. Digital images are generated which can be transferred via internal of external networks and processed and modified by various computer algorithms. Digital images allow for the direct measurement of biological structures and their functions. Accurate quantitative and qualitative information can be extracted. Two global categories of imaging modalities can be defined: Anatomical modalities depicting primarily information on morphology and functional modalities depicting primarily information on metabolism. The relationship of anatomical and functional information is of major interest for biological science and in particular for medical practice.

Various imaging modalities, including x-ray, CT, MR, PET, SPECT, ultrasound etc. are based on different physical principles thereby often containing complementary information. Each imaging modality possesses special attributes which may contribute to a better understanding of the physiology, abnormality or the disease. Many patients with signs and symptoms possibly related to a brain tumour undergo different imaging procedures including MRI, CT, SPECT and PET, each of them contributing specific information. CT and MRI provide complementary morphological information. For example MR optimally depicts brain tissue, but bony structures and calcifications are visualized better by CT. In addition many patients with brain tumours undergo radiation therapy necessitating a CT study for calculation of the dose distribution. Nuclear imaging modalities as SPECT and PET provide information about function (e.g. proliferation state with 201Tl or receptor status with somatostatin analogs) and metabolism (e.g. glucose uptake in 18FDG PET). Functional imaging has the capability to differentiate between metabolically active and inactive tissue corresponding to tumour or necrotic tissue.

Multiple 3D - image datasets are usually displayed with a light box side by side. For the clinician it is difficult to mentally integrate information from multiple diagnostic sources and construct a 3D - geometric relationship. Usually the radiologist extracts the useful data from the images and interprets it according to his knowledge. Whenever correlating information from multimodality studies from one patient is considered, the images should represent the same anatomy. However, since the same or different image sets acquired in the same subject may differ in scale, ori-

Table 1. Primarily morphological modalities

---
x-ray
Portal images
DSA (digital subtraction angiography)
CT (computed tomography)
CTA (computed tomography angiography)
MRI (magnetic resonance imaging)
US (ultrasound) including
Video images

Table 2. Primarily functional modalities

Scintigraphy
SPECT (single photon emission computed tomography) e.g. intra- and interictal SPECT
PET (positron emission tomography)
fMRI (functional MRI)
Doppler US
EEG (electro-encephalography)
EKG (electro-cardiography)
MEG (magnetoencephalography)
pMRI (perfusion MRI)
pCT (perfusion CT)

---

entation (angle) and position, an integration process is necessary in order to achieve a correct spatial alignment of all study modalities. This procedure is called registration. Recent advances in computer and software technology provide comprehensive capabilities for multimodal image fusion, which is useful in many medical applications in the whole body. Especially for applications in the brain for radiotherapy planning, anatomic mapping of cerebral function and tumour volume response to treatment image fusion was used successfully. After registration, a fusion step is required for the integrated display of the data involved [1]. Multimodality imaging is a synthesis of these different imaging datasets into a single composite image.

Besides multimodality registration monomodality registration is very important for verifying changes over time in order to monitor treatment and to get an idea about the biological features of various structures and pathologies, see figure E. In addition, differences between individuals and populations are investigated. In schizophrenia, for instance, subtle changes of certain structures of the brain in comparison to the normal population have been found using registration and quantitative volumetric measurements.

1 Methods of Medical Image Registration

Excellent survey of publications concerning medical imaging registration techniques were published by van der Elsen [2] Maintz and Viergever [1] and by Hanjal JH et al. [3]

Two different steps of integrating two or more images were defined: First, registration, bringing the modalities into spatial alignment and second, fusion for integrated display of the data. For medical applications usually 3D data is registered to 3D data, however it is also possible to register 2D to 3D data or coregister planar images. Applications of 2D-2D registration include comparison of different portal images at different times in order to evaluate and verify patient positioning during radiotherapy. An example of 2D - 3D registration is the matching of preoperative 3D - CT data with intraoperative fluoroscopy [4]. According to Maintz and Viergever the nature of registration basis can be classified extrinsic and intrinsic image-based registration and non-image-based registration. Extrinsic registration relies on external reference points that have to be introduced into the imaged space reliably in identical relationship to patient anatomy. These reference structures are either invasively or non-invasively attached to the patient. In contrast to extrinsic methods intrinsic methods rely on the patient image data only, thus allowing retrospective co-registration. A set of anatomical landmarks, segmented structures or the voxels itself are used for the registration process.

1.1 Extrinsic Methods

Invasive Extrinsic Methods The gold standard for registration accuracy are invasive stereotactic frames rigidly mounted on the patient's skull under local or general anaesthesia by means of pins or screws. These frames are usually applied for stereotactic neurosurgery, neurosurgical biopsies and radiosurgery. Conventional frames have to remain on the patient's skull in the time between the different image acquisitions and surgery, the patient often being anesthetized for a long time. According to this, invasive frames are limited by their short-term only application and not suitable for the purpose of (follow-up) multimodal image fusion.

Alternatively, invasive screws can be used as markers or as marker carriers [5], [6]. They provide an accuracy comparable to stereotactic frames. However, they may cause patient discomfort and should not be left in place over an extended period of time, thus application of invasive markers is not justified for diagnostic purposes solely.

Non-invasive Extrinsic Methods In order to overcome the drawbacks of invasive markers, adhesive, low cost skin markers may be applied [7], [8]. However, skin markers have several drawbacks including inaccuracies due to skin shift. If there are no clearly defined points on the skin (naevi, scars, etc.) for precise marker repositioning for the different scans, the markers have to remain on the patient's skin during the time between different scans. This problem may be solved by applying artificial ink landmarks to the skin.

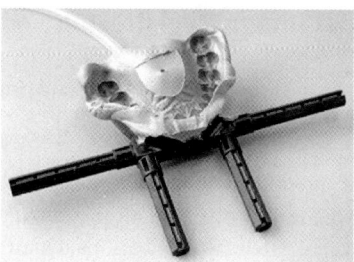

Fig. 1. The Vogele-Bale-Hohner mouthpiece with the vacuum area in the centre. The anterior and lateral rods may be used for the attachment of the reference frame and fixating arms.

The Laitinen stereoadapter [9] is mounted on the patient's head by means of two ear plugs, a nasion support and a connector plate over the vertex. The repositioning accuracy of this stereoadapter depends upon how tightly the support arms are braced between nasion, external auditory meati and vertex. Unfortunately, such rigid fixation-devices exert pressure on the external auditory canals and can cause patient discomfort and pain.

Attaching markers to mask-based fixation systems [10], [11], [12] is an interesting and viable method if one assumes high repositioning accuracy of the underlying anatomy. The accuracy of all mask based systems is however limited by movement of the underlying skin. The patient would also need to be fixated for each imaging procedure.

The systems of Hauser [13], the GTC localizer [14] the Banana Bar system [15] and the VBH mouthpiece [16] are devices based on a dental impression for repositioning an registration device on the patient: Hauser et al. fixate their referencing system on the patient by an upper dental cast, nasion and the external auditory meati. An attached N-box allows creates external points of reference. It is used for image-guided surgery in the ENT region. The GTC localizer [14] (Radionics Inc., Burlington, Mass., USA) is connected to the patient via an upper dental impression and a head support. Registration rods comparable to other commercially available invasive Stereotactic frames connected to the base ring of the frame provide precisely defined correlation points. The non-invasive relocatable Banana Bar (BB) fiducial marker system consists of a symmetrical U-shaped aluminum bar, sweeping backwards bilaterally along the head. It is held in place by actively biting on a dental impression of both maxillary and mandibular teeth.

The above mentioned devices that are based on dental impressions have two important drawbacks: First, they contain metallic components and therefore they are not suitable for MR exams, second the repositioning accuracy depends on the cooperation of the patient.

In 1994 our group has developed and patented the Vogele-Bale-Hohner (VBH) vacuum mouthpiece (Medical Intelligence Inc., Schwabmünchen, Germany) for computer-assisted ENT surgery and neurosurgery [17], [18]. The VBH mouthpiece is a simple, non-invasive and rigid device which does not contain any metallic com-

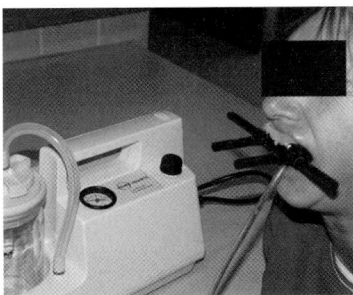

Fig. 2. Patient wearing the VBH mouthpiece: A tube connects the VBH mouthpiece with the vacuum pump. It fixates the mouthpiece on the upper dentition and allows for continuous monitoring of the positioning accuracy.

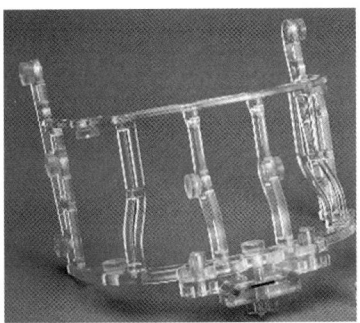

Fig. 3. The SIP-Lab Innsbruck frame contains 12 exchangeable spherical shaped markers. Depending on the imaging modality the respective markers are applied (glass beads for CT, nitrolingual capsules for MRI, ^{241}Am for SPECT, ^{18}F-FDG solution for PET)

ponents. Fabrication of the VBH mouthpiece takes 10 - 15 minutes and is fabricated prior to the initial scan. The form-stable impression material allows for repositioning accuracy of less than 1 mm [16]. In contrast to other systems a vacuum system fixates the VBH mouthpiece on the upper dentition of the patient and in addition, the vacuum pump guarantees continuous monitoring of the positioning accuracy. Recently we have developed a universal reference frame, the so-called SIP-Lab Innsbruck frame (Medical Intelligence Inc., Schwabmünchen, Germany), to be reproducibly mounted to the VBH mouthpiece. The SIP-Lab frame with its 12 markers is always and objectively in identical relationship to the cranium due to the negative pressure of the MP, irrespective of patient compliance.

Our phantom and patient study [19] showed that a high level of registration accuracy can be achieved despite the poor resolution of the scintigraphic images. In contrast to segmentation and voxel based registration methods the actual level of accuracy can be quantified by means of the RMSE value (root mean square error) as calculated by the software. The RMSE represents the mean distance between the matched paired-points after registration. Introduction of the mouthpiece with the frame takes additional 1 minute per CT/MR/SPECT/PET scan.

The localization error increases not only as a function of marker/ fiducial localization error (RSME) but also as the distance from the marker centroid to the point of interest increases [8]. Therefore the SIP-frame curves around the head with the most posterior markers located behind the ear. Since the markers are larger than the dimensions of a single voxel, defining their centre of mass in large magnification allows subvoxel registration accuracy [5]. It has to be noticed that the RMSE error is an indicator of the registration accuracy of the extrinsic reference points (frame), not the intrinsic anatomical structures. Our experiences however confirmed the results of a phantom study conducted at this institution, whereby fiducial (frame) and actual target registration error between CT/MR and CT/SPECT datasets correlated to under 1.5 mm.

We see the usefulness of this method mainly for registration of low resolution images such as SPECT and PET. The reference points on this frame grant completely objective registration using relatively simple and ubiquitous software, independent of a user's capability of defining anatomic landmarks or the varying limitations of more elaborate and costly algorithms. In addition we have developed an algorithm for automatic detection of the spherical markers of the reference frame on CT/MR/SPECT and PET, allowing a fully automatic extrinsic registration [20].

The limitations of the dental based reference systems are that accuracy of registration and repositioning is not reliable in edentulous patients. One important drawback of all extrinsic methods is the prospective character. This requires additional intrinsic methods that allow to performing the registration from the image content itself.

1.2 Intrinsic Methods

Anatomical Landmark-based Methods The simplest method is the use of anatomical landmarks. In the landmark-based registration method three or more appropriate, precisely definable landmarks or features are identified by the user or in an automatic fashion in the different image data sets and correlated to each other. Due to the good anatomical resolution, intrinsic registration methods work well for CT-CT, MR-MR and CT-MR fusion.

Our own experience is in accordance with that of other groups [3] that such anatomical landmarks can be co-registered to about 2-5 mm for CT and MRI. Such landmarks are however hard to define in SPECT/PET images.

It is often difficult to identify precisely the same anatomic features on two studies that reveal the anatomy in complementary fashion [21] requiring skill and practice of the user. The identification of the landmarks should be done or supervised by an experienced radiologist.

Surface-based Methods The "head-hat" method by Pelizzari et al. [22] relies on the segmentation of the skin surface from the different modalities. This method may yield gross misregistrations although the contours align perfectly due to identical

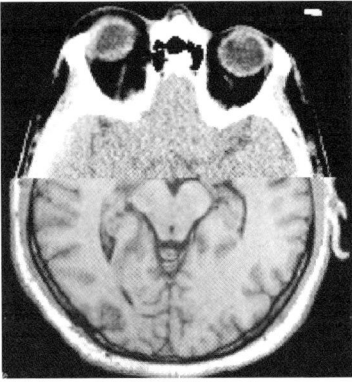

Fig. 4. Visual inspection of CT-MRI registration of the brain based on mutual information algorithm shows a satisfactory result.

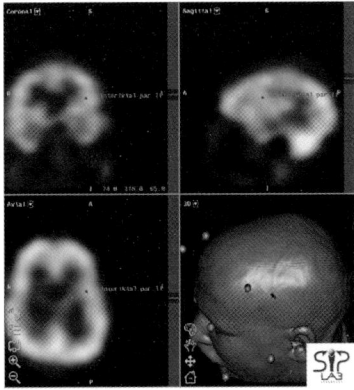

Fig. 5. Due to the low resolution SPECT images appear very blurry and it is very difficult to define (precise) anatomical landmarks as demonstrated in these axial, sagittal and coronal reformatted interictal SPECT data of the brain.

axes of symmetry. Different imaging modalities can also provide substantially different image contrast between corresponding surfaces. The registration accuracy is limited to the accuracy of the segmentation step which is especially problematic in SPECT/PET images.

1.3 Voxel-property Based Methods

Voxel property-based registration methods [23],[24] rely on the image grey values without prior segmentation, using the full image content for the registration process. In most approaches the registration is performed automatically. The voxel property-based or mutual-information based registration methods are not influenced by segmentation errors or subjective determination of anatomical landmarks. Comparisons of mutual information based registration with external marker based registration of the brain as part of the retrospective evaluation project performed at the Vanderbilt University, TN, USA showed subvoxel accuracy of CT to MR and PET to MR. It is highly robust and does not require segmentation or definition of landmarks. Therefore it is very user-friendly and useful for daily clinical routine. However, especially in extra-cranial regions problems related to the intrinsic based registration method may occur, see figure I. In addition, the quality of registration is also influenced by the resolution of the images, modality specific image degradations and artefacts. Due to the intrinsic selective uptake of tracers only in areas with altered metabolism, SPECT images do not sufficiently depict the anatomy. For this reason precise, internal anatomical markers, precise surfaces and comparable voxels are lacking so that image fusion based on intrinsic information may fail.

The result of CT-MR registration can be visually checked by the naked eye. Registration results seem somewhat more satisfying in methods involving SPECT and PET images because the blurry nature of the images seems to allow a larger displacement. The image resolution should not be used to formulate a clinically relevant level of accuracy: SPECT-to-MR or PET-to-MR registration may even require higher accuracy than some instances of CT-to-MR registration, even though the smaller error is more easily assessed by the naked eye in the latter case. The actual level of accuracy is still unknown in many applications, and cannot be quantified accurately, even by the clinicians involved.

Especially in cases where scintigraphic images are implemented in neurosurgery, radiotherapy or other therapeutic interventions high precision of co-registration is paramount.

All the above mentioned algorithms assume the image datasets as rigid bodies.

2 Non-image Based Registration

2.1 Combined PET-CT or SPECT-CT Scanners

Non-image based registration is possible if the coordinate systems of different scanners are calibrated to each other. Combined PET/CT or SPECT-CT scanners provide spatially registered images from the two modalities acquired in a single imaging session.

2.2 CT-US Fusion

Another example is a navigated ultrasound system where the ultrasound probe is tracked by a 3D -localization system, the patient being immobilized in the CT-or MR-scanner. Due to a calibration of the ultrasound system with the coordinates of the scanner a real-time registration and fusion of ultrasound images with reconstructed CT/MR images can be performed [25].

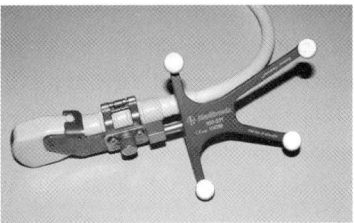

Fig. 6. A dynamic reference frame with 4 reflective markers is mounted to the SonoNav ultrasound probe. The reflective markers are detected by the cameras of the navigation system, which calculated the actual position of the ultrasound probe in 3D space with respect to the patient.

In the SIP-Lab Innsbruck a different approach is performed: The patient is scanned in the CT/MR/SPECT/PET with artifical markers attached to the patient, the BodyFix or the SIP-Lab frame. The dataset is sent to the navigation system. The patient is registered in the laboratory or in the OR using the navigation system. A video signal of the tracked ultrasound probe (SONONav, Medtronic, USA) is sent to the navigation system and the navigation system reconstructs the respective planes of the CT/MR/SPECT/PET in real time, thus the actual ultrasound image can be superimposed to the pre-operative scan datasets.

The weighting of the ultrasound image over the other modalities can be adjusted via mouse-controlled sliders. This technology has originally been developed for the compensation of brain shift during neurosurgical interventions. However it can be used in the whole body using various immobilization and registration devices.

3 Routine Application of Image Fusion for Diagnosis and Interventions at the Interdisciplinary Stereotactic Intervention- and Planning Laboratory (SIP-Lab)

A few years ago the optical based Treon navigation system (Medtronic Inc., Louisville, U.S.A.) was installed at our interdisciplinary laboratory for image-guided neuro-, ENT- and orthopaedic- surgery. The software module "Cranial 4" is part of the Treon navigation system. It allows for synergistic simultaneous fusion of any combination of CT/MR/SPECT/PET data based on paired-point matching of extrinsic markers or intrinsic (anatomical) markers. In addition, a mutual based fully automatic algorithm for fusion of CT/MR/SPECT/PET data is available.

3.1 The "Cranial 4" Multimodality Software:

The CT/MR/SPECT/PET studies respective of each patient are transferred to the Treon via hospital own intranet. The Cranial 4 multimodality software allows the

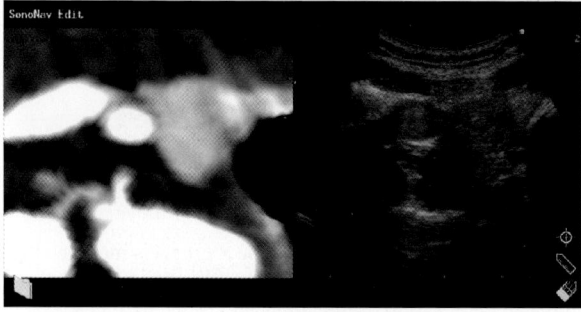

Fig. 7. Sononavigation in the neck area: Left image: reformatted CT according to the realtime-ultrasound image. Right image: 50 % superposition of the real-time ultrasound with the real-time reformatted CT.

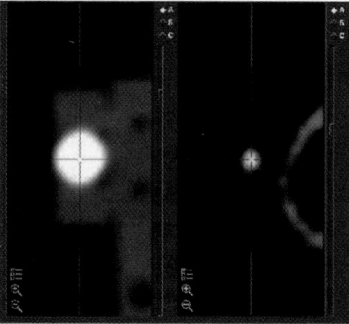

Fig. 8. The centres of the external landmarks in the CT data (left) and SPECT data (right) are selected in the highest possible magnification.

user to correlate up to 10 different image sets of one patient and to display and review the correlated images.

The registration procedure is a one-to-one mapping between the reference and the working image set ensuring that the same anatomical point in both images corresponds to each other. Image fusion software process starts with loading of the reference CT scan, which remains the base standard for fusion with MR/SPECT/PET since it is free of distortion artefacts. After preview and verification of the images the CT dataset is set as a reference, the following CT/MR/SPECT datasets as working image sets. The Cranial 4 software is capable of two different image registration methods; both are rigid-model based:

1. Paired-point matching
   The registration is performed manually by selecting a minimum of 4 clearly defined corresponding fiducials or anatomical landmarks on both, the reference and the working dataset. The landmarks are selected by pointing-and-clicking the mouse cursor within the image in the highest possible magnification.

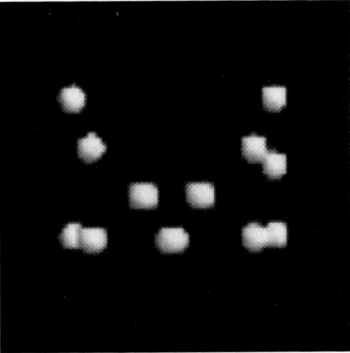

Fig. 9. A 3D reconstruction of the ^{241}Am markers on the SIP Lab Innsbruck frame based on SPECT data.

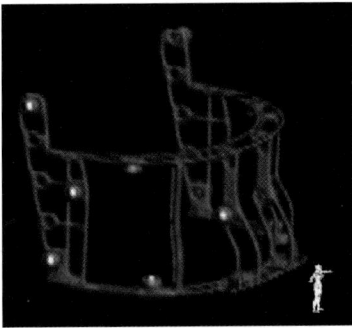

Fig. 10. A 3D reconstruction of the reference frame with the glass bead markers based on helical CT data.

Using the SIP Lab Innsbruck frame 4 - 12 spherical fiducials (external markers) are selected for each registration process

When manually registering two data sets, registration accuracy is calculated by the software as the root square mean error (RSME) which is the mean distance of the respective frame-reference points in the two data sets.

2. Voxel-intensity based algorithm
   The fully automatic voxel-intensity algorithm implemented in the Cranial 4 workstation is based on the use of the general notion of mutual information. It allows us to import and co-register the previous CT/MR images, which were obtained without the frame, with the actual multimodal datasets, which are obtained with the frame.

3.2 Fusion / Display

Once the image set has been registered the Cranial 4 software provides a variety of tools which enable the user to quantitatively and qualitatively compare the registered image sets. The software enables the user to combine the registered image sets by using the blend mode for visual comparison of results.

In this manner, each image modality can be displayed with the others as a combined level of reference and working pixel intensities in three planes (axial, coronal, sagittal). The threshold levels of all image sets as well as the weighting of one modality over the other can be adjusted via mouse-controlled sliders allowing quick visualization of any region in any magnification in three planes (axial, coronal, sagittal). Using interactive linked cursors a pixel to pixel correspondence can be evaluated. Up to ten further previously registered studies, be it CT, MRI or functional imaging studies (SPECT/PET), can then be uploaded and compared to each other individually.

4 Implementation of Multimodal Image Data into Image-guided ENT and Neurosurgery

Image-guided surgery may be performed on the basis of the multimodal datasets. The tip of the pointer is displayed in real-time on re-sliced 2D and 3D images. A transformation of the coordinate system associated with the pre-operative datasets and the coordinate system of the 3D - localizer is achieved. For such a link structures that are visible on the imaged data and that can be detected by the 3D - localizer must exist. For many neurosurgical procedures high registration accuracies are required which - according to our own experiences in more than hundred ENT cases - cannot be achieved with simple anatomical paired-point matching. Mutual information based registration algorithms can - as a matter of course - not be used for registration of imaged space to physical space. Some groups use surface based algorithms by rendering the skin surface of the 3D object and touching at least 30 points on the patient or, alternatively, using a laser to render a 3D - surface of the real patient. As discussed above the accuracy of these methods are sensitive to tissue shift and depend on correct rendering of the skin surface. In addition, an irregular shape of the surface is paramount for an accurate registration. In order to achieve higher degrees of accuracy reliable extrinsic reference points are necessary.

Invasive markers are accurate, but they are cumbersome for the patient and the surgeon. For most image-guided neurosurgical procedures a prospective registration based on skin fiducials is performed, even though this method is sensitive to soft tissue shift which may result in deviations. An additional preoperative MRI has to be acquired, with the skin markers attached to the patient. We routinely use the reference points on the SIP-Lab Innsbruck frame for image-guided neurosurgery.

1. Image Fusion and image-guided surgery in the cranial area

Multimodality Registration in Daily Clinical Practice 177

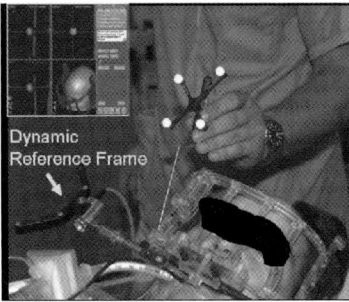

Fig. 11. Image-guided neurosurgery using the VBH mouthpiece: The dynamic reference frame and the SIP-Lab frame are attached to the mouthpiece. The markers on the frame are indicated by the probe of the navigation system and the corresponding fiducials are selected on the 3D-image dataset.

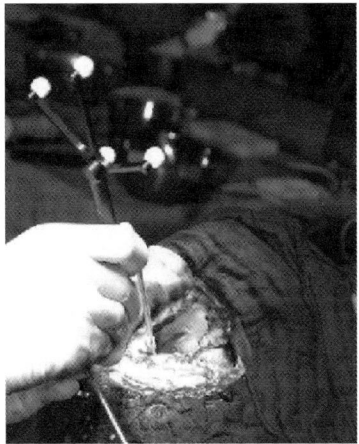

Fig. 12. After registration the reference frame is removed and the surgeon can use the pointer to navigate during neurosurgery.

In patients with intact dentition of the upper jaw a VBH mouthpiece is made at initial presentation of a patient presenting with symptoms suspicious of a cranial tumor [18]. The initial 3D CT/ MRI /SPECT /PET data sets can then be registered and used for frameless stereotactic neurosurgery and/or radiation -planning and -treatment [26], [27] as well as brachytherapy applications [28], reducing the need for additional scans as the patient proceeds from department to department. Previous anatomical and functional datasets are registered to the current data by voxel-based algorithms or, in selected cases, by choosing intrinsic landmarks.

In edentulous patients the different CT- and MR- and PET- datasets are registered to each other by mutual information algorithms or, in some cases, by

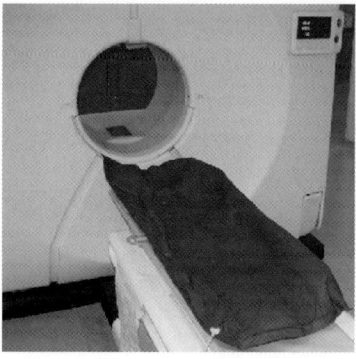

Fig. 13. Individual mattress for CT-PET fusion of the body.

selecting clearly defined anatomical landmarks. For image-guided surgery an additional MRI scan of the patient with skin fiducials is performed.

2. Extra-cranial Image-fusion

All the above mentioned algorithms assume the image datasets as rigid bodies. The result of extra-cranial image fusion highly depends on the positioning of the patient in the various scanners. In addition, different filling of the bladder and the gut as well as differences in breathing may cause big deviations (up to 5 cm, experience by the author). The most important reason is the different respiration patterns during the different scan acquisitions. Frequently we are asked to fuse image datasets in a retrospective manner. Retrospective image fusion of CT/MR/SPECT/PET datasets using mutual information based algorithms provides sometimes disastrous results which cannot be applied for diagnostic purposes. In these cases we try to use anatomical landmarks. Every organ near the diaphragm has to be matched separately.

For precise fusion identical positioning and fixation is required. This can be performed by immobilizing the patient in the scanners with an individually formed vacuum mattress. Depending on the type of imaging the respective external markers are attached to the fixation system.

4.1 Procedure

An individual mattress from the patient is formed by the radiation technician prior to the image acquisition.

This takes about 5-10 minutes. The vacuum mattress is stored in the SIP-Lab. For every imaging acquisition (CT/PET/SPECT) the patient is repositioned into the vacuum mattress and the respective markers are attached to the mattress at identical positions.

We use 5 markers per region (thorax, head/neck or abdomen). During the PET and SPECT acquisition the patients breathe normally. For the CT scan the patient has to expire slightly and keep his breath during the scan. In most scanners respiratory triggering for PET and SPECT is not available. Thus the resulting information is

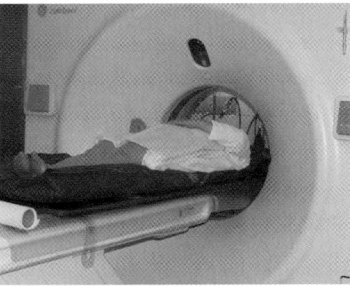

Fig. 14. For imaging acquisition the patient is repositioned into the vacuum mattress and the respective markers are attached to the mattress at identical positions.

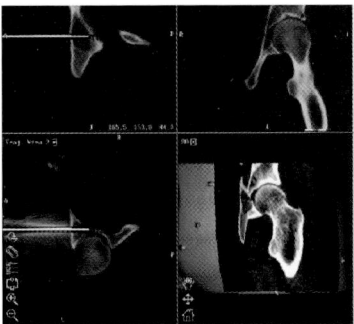

Fig. 15. Evaluating the accuracy of an image guided puncture for radiofrequency ablation of a hypernephroma metastasis in the right acetabulum: The intraoperative CT is fused with the pre-operative planning dataset and the actual position of the instrument is superimposed to the planned path.

a sum of the information provided by different respiratory positions. By our breathing protocol an optimal correlation between the functional data and the anatomical data can be achieved, see figure G and H. Using this respiratory triggering the lung and the organs in the upper abdomen are in a similar position according to the "mean position" during the PET/SPECT acquisition. The same breathing protocol should also be used in combined PET/SPECT - CT scanners. The different datasets are sent to the Treon navigation system and registered to each other by means of paired-point matching.

4.2 Examples of Clinical Applications of Image Fusion that are Routinely Performed by the SIP-Lab Innsbruck

1. Diagnostic work-up
   In most cases image fusion is used in the diagnostic investigation of a variety of pathologic conditions including tumors, inflammations etc. Fusion of SPECT and CT is routinely used in the investigation of hyperparathyroidism and neuro-

endocrine neoplasm. Fusion of PET with MR/CT is routinely performed in patients with cancer.
2. Epilepsy - Detection of the anatomic origin of the seizure activity
   a) Fusion of MR - PET - ictal and interictal SPECT, see figure F and K
   For localization of the origin of the seizure different imaging data are available, all providing different information. For epilepsy patients it is important to have conclusive diagnostic information concerning the origin of the seizure. In patients with a conclusive localization the respective brain area is resected. In a high percentage of epilepsy cases the origin of the seizure is located in the hippocampus. The so-called hippocampal sclerosis can be visualized by MRI and must be confirmed by image fusion with the functional imaging (PET/SPECT) prior to surgery.
   In addition data from the EEG and videomonitoring are important for the therapeutic decision. In some cases structural abnormalities in other brain areas are responsible for the disease. These lesions may also be detected by MRI and must be confirmed by functional imaging.
   b) Detection of the focus of seizure activity based on the EEG
   In the remaining cases the MRI does not reveal any pathology or anatomical abnormality the decision for surgery is very difficult. The EEG electrodes can be replaced by markers visible in MRI. A 3D - reconstruction of the brain and the skin markers are performed visualizing the region of the brain being responsible for the seizure activity.
   c) Fusion of two different 3D - objects from different image acquisitions:
   If the fusion of anatomical data and functional data and the other neurological examinations do not provide enough information about localization of the seizure origin invasive electrodes are implanted directly on the brain surface or via the foramen ovale inside the basal cisterns. For precise lesion localization it is important to know the actual location of the different electrodes with respect to the brain surface. Therefore two 3D - models have to be reconstructed, one 3D reconstruction of the brain surface and one of the electrodes. A post-operative CT scan is obtained to reconstruct the electrodes. However due to the artefacts of the electrodes it is not possible to reconstruct the brain surface with sufficient quality. Thus the post-operative 3D - CT dataset is matched with the pre-operative 3D MR dataset. A 3D reconstruction of the brain surface of the MR is then superimposed to the 3D - reconstruction of the electrodes of the postoperative CT. By this means 3D - volume images indicate the positions of subdural and trigeminal electrodes with respect to the brain surface, see figure D.
   d) Subtraction of inter-ictal from ictal SPECT data (between and during seizures).
   In some patients the acquisition of a SPECT between and during the seizures is required. By using a subtraction algorithm the active focus remains. By fusing this active focus with an MR scan the anatomical localization of this focus can be visualized.

3. Radiotherapy planning
   CT is needed for calculation of the dose distribution, MR is required for precise definition of the treatment volume due to better outlining of the tumour tissue. Accurate CT-MR-SPECT-PET image registration allows for precise definition of active tumour tissue to be irradiated.
4. Follow-up: verification of treatment
   Monomodality registration by comparison of pre-and post-intervention images (after radiation therapy, chemotherapy, surgery etc.) is an interesting tool for growth monitoring and treatment verification.
5. Evaluation of accuracy of image guided punctures
   During an image guided puncture an intraoperative CT or MR can be obtained. This dataset can be fused with the pre-operative planning dataset and the actual position of the biopsy needle, the driller or the drill-hole can be superimposed to the planned path.
6. Sono-navigation
   The Sono-navigation tool can be used for diagnostic purposes. We currently use it for the comparison of CT, MIBI-SPECT and ultrasound in the diagnosis of parathyroid adenoma. Ultrasound can also be used as an intraoperative real-time imaging tool to compensate brain shift.

4.3 Conclusion

This article focuses on the methods used in daily clinical practice by the authors. Currently we use only rigid of affine transformations. For further information on other registration algorithms in other medical fields see the paper by Lavallee [25] and the review paper by Maintz and Viergever [1]. Elastic deformation algorithms are currently developed and are very interesting for inter-subject and atlas registration. Advances in imaging and computer technology should increase and optimize the extraction and quantification of useful inherent information and the application of this information for patient treatment. Effective visualization, synthesis, extraction and analysis of fused 3D biomedical images will be enhanced by continuing improvement of current methods. Multimodality image fusion provides synergistic information about the different imaging data, which might result in a better interpretation of the total imaging data. Hopefully this may result in a more effective diagnosis and treatment of disease.

5 Acknowledgment

All the nuclear medicine images were acquired at the Department of Nuclear Medicine in Innsbruck. The following persons are involved in the development and/or clinical applications of the SIP-Lab image fusion technology:

Department of Radiology Innsbruck (Prof. Dr. W. Jaschke): P. Kovacs, T. Lang, M. Knoflach, C. Hinterleithner, W. Jaschke

Department of Nuclear Medicine (Prof. Dr. I. Virgolini): Moncayo, Donnemiller, Gabriel, Heute, Kendler

Department of Neurosurgery (Prof. Dr. K. Twerdy): Eisner, Burtscher, Fiegele, Gabl, Ortler

Department of Orthopaedics (Prof. Dr. W. Krismer): Rachbauer

Department of Radiotherapy (Prof. Dr. P. Lukas): Sweeney, Nevinny, Seydl

Department of Neurology (Prof. Dr. W. Poewe): Trinka, Stockhammer, Unterberger, Dobesberger

Department of Surgery (Prof. Dr. E. Magreiter): Prommegger, Profanter

References

1. J. Maintz and M. Viergever: A survey of medical image registration, Medical Image Analysis **2**, pp 1-36, (1998)
2. P. A. van den Elsen and M. A. Viergever: Medical Image Matching - a review with classification, IEEE Computer Graphics and Applications **12**, pp 26-39, (2004)
3. J. H. Hanjal, D. J. Hawkes and D. Hill: Medical Image Registration, Biomedical Engineering Series (2004)
4. J. Weese, G. P. Penney, P. Desmedt, et al: Voxel-based 2-D/3-D registration of fluoroscopy images and CT scans for image-guided surgery, IEEE Trans Inf Technol Biomed **1**, pp 284-93, (1997)
5. C. R. Maurer Jr., J. M. Fitzpatrick, M. Y. Wang, et al.: Registration of head volume images using implantable fiducial markers, IEEE Trans Med Imaging **16**, pp 477–62, (1997)
6. C. Kremser, C. Plangger, R. Bosecke, et al: Image registration of MR and CT images using a frameless fiducial marker system, Magn Reson Imaging **15**, pp 579-89, (1997)
7. N. T. Evans: Combining imaging techniques, Clin Phys Physiol Meas **11**, pp 97-102, (1990)
8. S. J. Zinreich, S. A. Tebo, D. M. Long, et al: Frameless stereotaxic integration of CT imaging data: accuracy and initial applications, Radiology **188**, pp 735-42, (1993)
9. H. Hirschberg and O. J. Kirkeby: Interactive image directed neurosurgery: patient registration employing the Laitinen stereo-adapter, Minim Invasive Neurosurg **39**, pp 105-7, (1996)
10. T. Greitz, M. Bergstrom, J. Boethius, et al: Head fixation system for integration of radiodiagnostic and therapeutic procedures, Neuroradiology **19**, pp 1-6, (1980)
11. M. Bergstrom, J. Boethius, L. Eriksson, et al: Head fixation device for reproducible position alignment in transmission CT and positron emission tomography, J Comput Assist Tomogr **5**, pp 136-41, (1981)
12. M. N. Pilipuf, J. C. Goble and N. F. Kassell: A noninvasive thermoplastic head immobilization system. Technical note, J Neurosurg **82**, pp 1082-5, (1995)
13. R. Hauser, B. Westermann and R. Probst: Noninvasive tracking of patient's head movements during computer-assisted intranasal microscopic surgery, Laryngoscope **107**, pp 494-9, (1997)
14. S. S. Gill, D. G. Thomas, A. P. Warrington, et al: Relocatable frame for stereotactic external beam radiotherapy, Int J Radiat Oncol Biol Phys **20**, pp 599-603, (1991)
15. M. A. Howard III, M. B. Dobbs, T. M. Simonson, et al: A noninvasive, reattachable skull fiducial marker system. Technical note, J Neurosurg **83**, pp 372-6, (1995)

16. A. Martin, R. J. Bale, M. Vogele, et al: Vogele-Bale-Hohner mouthpiece: registration device for frameless stereotactic surgery, Radiology **208**, pp 261-5, (1998)
17. R. J. Bale, M. Vogele, W. Freysinger, et al.: Minimally invasive head holder to improve the performance of frameless stereotactic surgery, Laryngoscope **107**, pp 373-7, (1997)
18. R. J. Bale, J. Burtscher, W. Eisner, et al.: Computer-assisted neurosurgery by using a noninvasive vacuum-affixed dental cast that acts as a reference base: another step toward a unified approach in the treatment of brain tumors, J Neurosurg **93**, pp 208-13, (2000)
19. R. A. Sweeney, R. J. Bale, R. Moncayo, et al.: Multimodality cranial image fusion using external markers applied via a vacuum mouthpiece and a case report, Strahlenther Onkol **179**, pp 254-60, (2003)
20. M. Capek, R. Wegenkittl, A. Koenig, W. Jaschke, R. A. Sweeney, and R. J. Bale: Multimodal Volume Registration based on spherical markers, Conference proceedings of the 9th International Conference in Central Europe on Computer Graphics, Visualization and Computer Vision **1**, pp 17-24, (2001)
21. D. N. Levin, C. A. Pelizzari, G. T. Chen, et al: Retrospective geometric correlation of MR, CT, and PET images, Radiology **169**, pp 817-23, (1988)
22. C. A. Pelizzari, G. T. Chen, D. R. Spelbring, et al.: Accurate three-dimensional registration of CT, PET, and/or MR images of the brain, J Comput Assist Tomogr **13**, pp 20-6, (1989)
23. W. M. Wells III, P. Viola, H. Atsumi, et al.: Multi-modal volume registration by maximization of mutual information, Med Image Anal **1**, pp 35-51, (1996)
24. C. Studholme, D. L. Hill, and D. J. Hawkes: Automated 3-D registration of MR and CT images of the head, Med Image Anal **1**, pp 163-75, (1996)
25. S. Lavallee, P. Cinquin, R. Szeliski, et al.: Building a hybrid patient's model for augmented reality in surgery: a registration problem, Comput Biol Med **25**, pp 149-64, (1995)
26. R. Sweeney, R. J. Bale, M. Vogele, et al.: Repositioning accuracy: comparison of a noninvasive head holder with thermoplastic mask for fractionated radiotherapy and a case report, Int J Radiat Oncol Biol Phys **41**, pp 475-83, (1998)
27. R. A. Sweeney, R. J. Bale, T. Auberger, et al: A simple and non-invasive vacuum mouthpiece-based head fixation system for high precision radiotherapy, Strahlenther Onkol **177**, pp 43-7, (2001)
28. R. J. Bale, W. Freysinger, A. R. Gunkel, et al.: Head and neck tumors: fractionated frameless stereotactic interstitial brachytherapy-initial experience, Radiology **214**, pp 591-5, (2004)

Colour Images

Clarenz et al., Henn et al., Weickert et al., and Bale

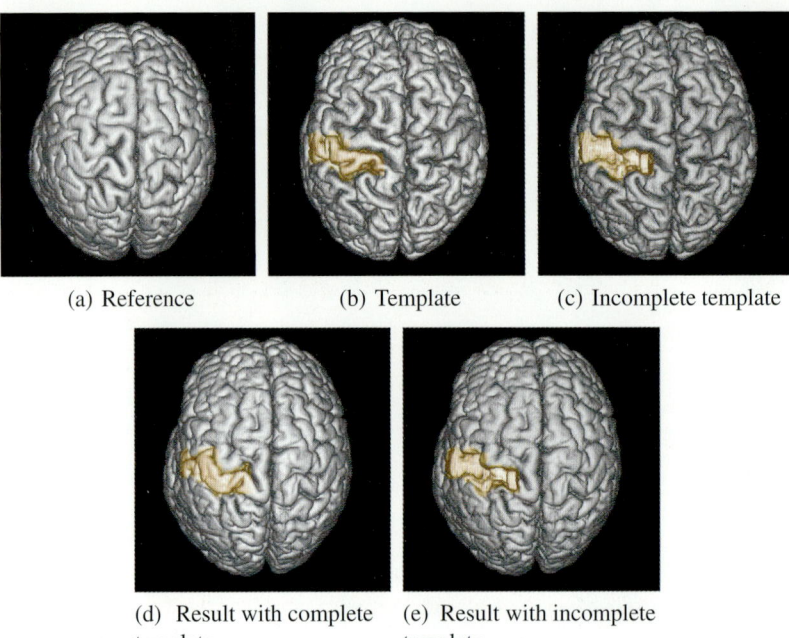

(a) Reference (b) Template (c) Incomplete template

(d) Result with complete template (e) Result with incomplete template

Fig. A. Here surface renderings of the reference, template and result brains are shown. The brains are displayed from top view, slightly tilted to the right. The frontal part of the brain is always at the top of the image. The corresponding mask are projected onto the surface. Figure (d) shows the result for the registration with the complete template. Figure (e) shows the result with the incomplete template, when a lesion mask is provided.

Colour Images 187

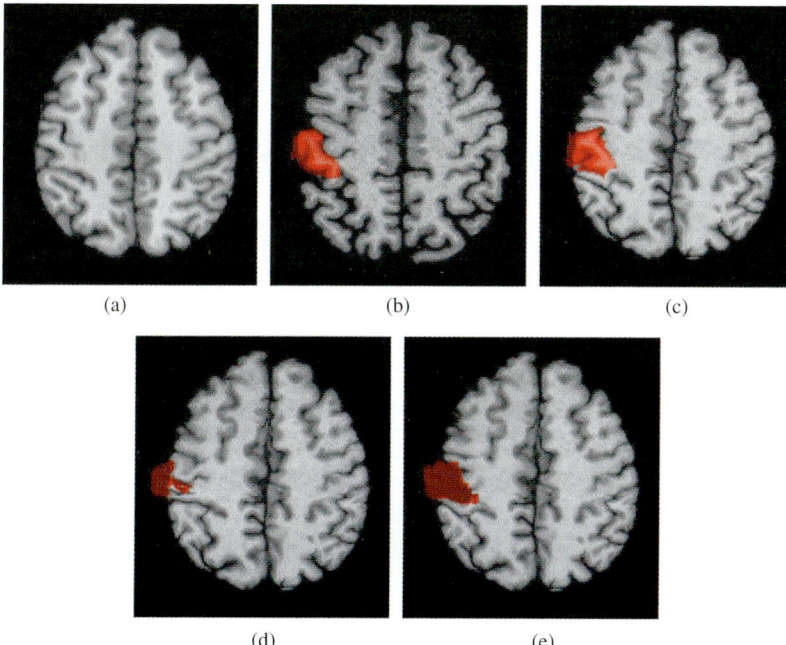

Fig. B. All subfigures show the same horizontal slice in different brains. Figure (a) shows the reference and figure (b) the template with the overlayed lesion mask. Results for the three different registration are shown in figure (c)-(e). The first one is the result for the registration with the complete template. Then comes the registration with the incomplete template without the lesion mask (d) and with the lesion mask (e).

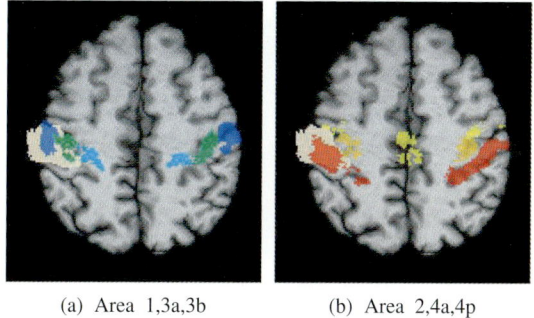

(a) Area 1,3a,3b   (b) Area 2,4a,4p

Fig. C. Here a horizontal slice of the registered brain, overlayed with the lesion mask and probability maps for a number of cortical areas, is shown. The colors for the cortical areas are: 1–blue, 3a–light blue, 3b–green, 2–red, 4a–yellow, 4p–orange.

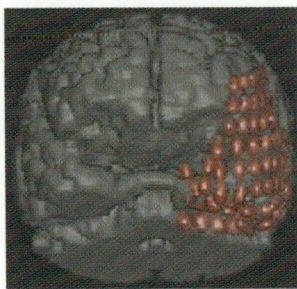

Fig. D. Fusion of the 3D-surface of the brain from the pre-operative MRI and the 3D-reconstruction of the electrodes from the post-operative CT.

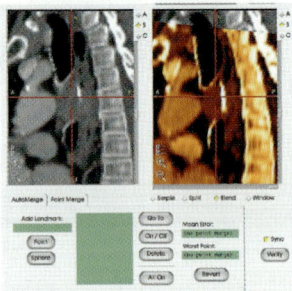

Fig. E. Sagittal views after fusion of a CT of a patient with oesophageal carcinoma before (left) and after (right) chemotherapy. Monomodality registration allows for precise monitoring of the growth/treatment success in 3 dimensions.

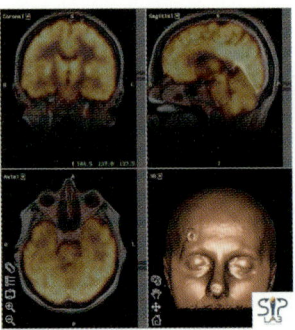

Fig. F. Patient with right sided hippocampal sclerosis in the anatomical MRI and decrease of activation in the functional PET (blend mode 50 %).

Colour Images 189

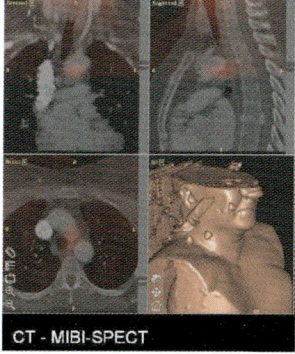

Fig. G. Fusion of ^{99m}Tc-SPECT and CT in a patient with primary hyperparathyroidism showing an activation in the mediastinum which corresponds to a soft tissue mass visible in the CT scan. Surgery confirmed an atypically located parathyroid adenoma.

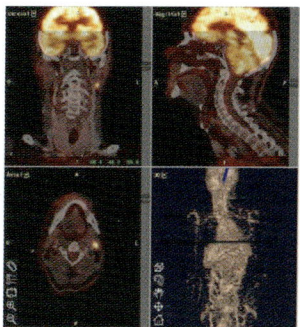

Fig. H. Follow-up CT-PET image fusion in a patient with Hodgkin lymphoma of the stomach reveals an additional pathological lymphnode in the neck, which was initially not detected in the CT scan.

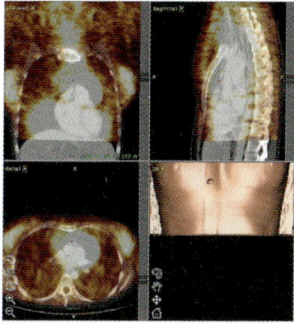

Fig. I. Visual inspection shows a disastrous result after retrospective CT-PET fusion of the thorax using mutual information algorithm requiring additional registration based on anatomical landmarks.

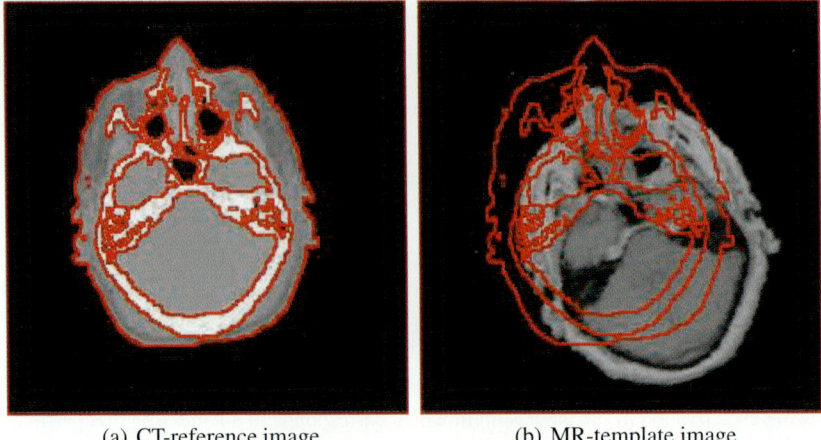

(a) CT-reference image (b) MR-template image

Fig. J. Example for a multi-modal image registration problem: computer tomography (CT)–magnetic resonance imaging (MRI). Both images are presented with superimposed reference contour.

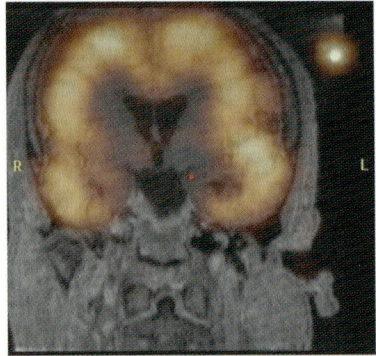

Fig. K. depicts coronal reconstruction of a fusion (blend mode 50%) of MRI and ^{123}I-Iomazenil - SPECT in a patient with left temporal lobe epilepsy (red dot).

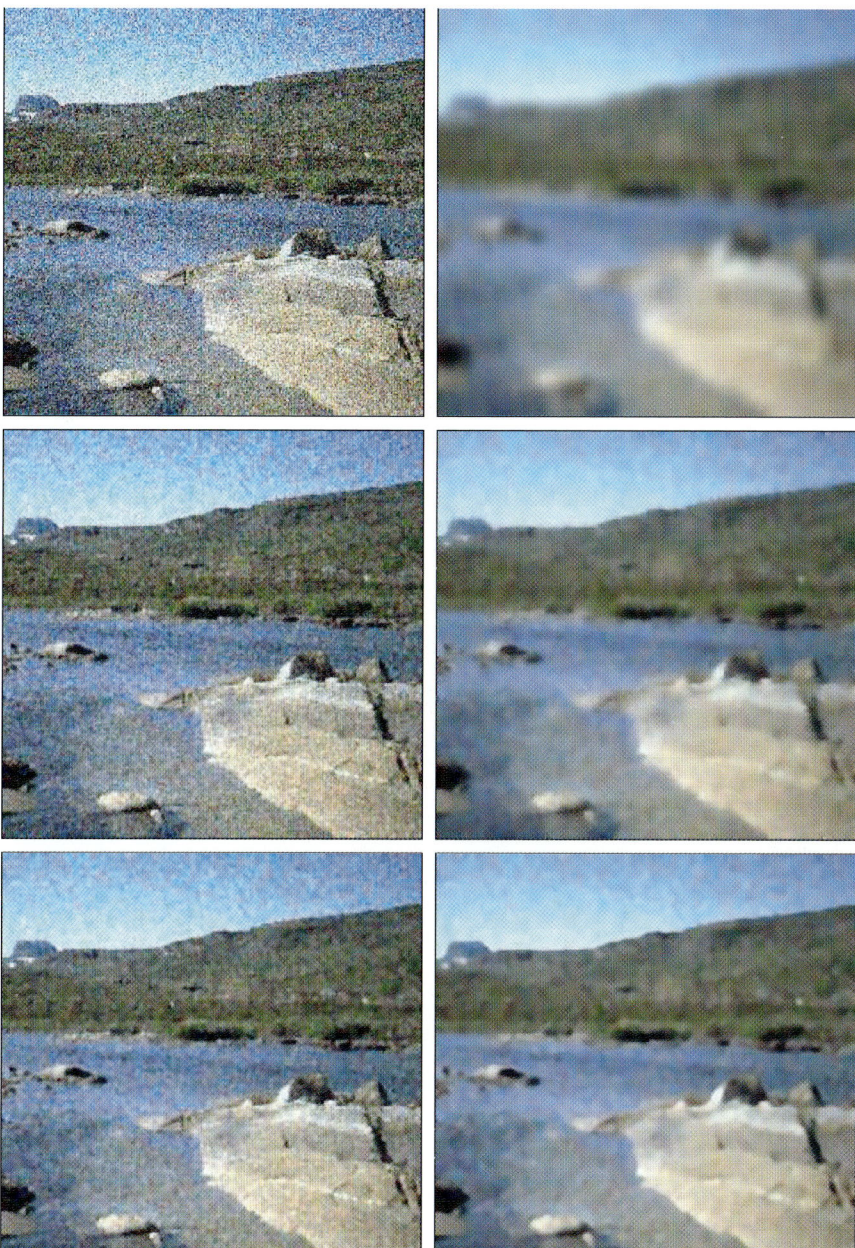

Fig. L. Diffusion filtering of colour images. *(a) Top left:* Noisy color image. *(b) Top right:* Homogeneous diffusion. *(c) Middle left:* Linear isotropic diffusion. *(d) Middle right:* Linear anisotropic diffusion. *(e) Bottom left:* Nonlinear isotropic diffusion. *(f) Bottom right:* Nonlinear anisotropic diffusion. From [89].

Printing: Krips bv, Meppel
Binding: Stürtz, Würzburg